THE WAVEFORM MODEL
OF VOWEL PERCEPTION
AND PRODUCTION

THE WAVEFORM MODEL OF VOWEL PERCEPTION AND PRODUCTION

MICHAEL A. STOKES

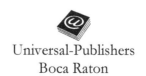

Universal-Publishers
Boca Raton

The Waveform Model of Vowel Perception and Production

Universal-Publishers
Boca Raton, Florida • USA
2009

ISBN-10: 1-59942-888-1
ISBN-13: 978-1-59942-888-8

www.universal-publishers.com

CONTENTS

ACKNOWLEDGEMENTS

Special thanks to Dr. John Mullennix for his technical support and talker database. Our discussions and his critical feedback have been invaluable in this effort. Early support from Dr. Brian Scott also came at a needed point in time. Finally, this study would not have been possible without the love and support of my parents and family.

The visual cues contained within raw complex waveforms have led to a unique method of organizing the vowel space. Formant relationships are used to categorize and distinguish each vowel, with the categorization method associating a formant frequency with a specific articulatory gesture. The method of categorization also provides an explanation for vowel perceptual errors identified in human and computer vowel perception experiments. As a test of the model described in this book, formant frequency measurements were obtained from the mid point of the vowels produced by 20 males (524 total vowels), with the vowels subsequently identified using the features of the Waveform Model in perceptual experiments. Results showed 93.9% vowel identification accuracy across the 20 males using the original method of calculating the relationship of F1 to F0 in Experiment I, with the few errors observed accounted for within the model. Changing the method of calculating the relationship of F1 to F0 in Experiment II produced 97.7% accuracy across the same vowels tested in Experiment I. The focus here will be to introduce and describe the unique concepts of the Waveform Model, and to describe the experimental evidence that supports the model.

AUTHOR'S BACKGROUND

The author has extensive experience analyzing over 15,000 speech waveforms, with this work exhibited in a number of past presentations and published work. The first significant project involved analyzing speech produced in noise (Summers et al., 1988), followed by analysis of speech produced under conditions of cognitive workload (Summers et al., 1989). The author's next presentation represented the initial research showing that vowels can be identified from visual inspection of the waveforms of vowels (Stokes, 1996). To extend this work, the research was replicated with two additional male talkers and one female talker (Stokes, 2001). Beyond the identification of vowels from visual analysis of waveforms, the identification of a talker was achieved from waveforms (i.e., voiceprints, similar to the use of fingerprints, Stokes, 2002). Altogether, this work is innovative in its reliance on waveform displays as an analysis tool, and has contributed to the overall understanding of speech perception in a number of environments.

Since 1998, the author has been employed as a computer programmer working on a number of international business applications. The programming and database skills utilized in these positions have led to the ability to perform the experiments and analyze the data in great detail. The internet programming experience also allowed the author to post early versions of the model under the working name MAS Model of Vowel Perception and Production on the internet in December of 1998. The feedback obtained from researchers in the field proved to be valuable as the work progressed to the level it is now with 97.7% vowel identification accuracy across 20 male talkers.

CHAPTER 1

BACKGROUND

The waveform model is based on combinations of cues originally identified from the visual display of raw complex waveforms. An individual formant from a vowel possesses characteristics of a sine wave at a particular frequency and amplitude. A raw complex waveform is the single wave created from the combination of vowels' individual formants. Spectrograms are a useful tool for acoustic-phonetic analysis of formants because they separate individual formants making detailed analysis of vowels' components possible. However, the interactions of the components are lost, and a great deal of effort has been spent theorizing about how the individual formants interact to give a vowel its quality. Unlike spectrogram displays, raw complex waveforms maintain the interactive quality of the formants.

There has been a fair amount of success in visually identifying speech sounds from spectrogram displays (Cole, Rudnicky, & Zue, 1979; Cole, R., and Zue, V., 1980). However, there was no such success in identifying speech sounds from raw complex waveforms until the presentations by Stokes (Stokes, 1996, 2001). In fact, it has been taught for some time that "[i]t is not possible to look at the waveform of an utterance and say what sounds occurred" (Ladefoged, 1982, p. 168). Although this statement is somewhat dated, it is still being taught. There are only limited descriptions of the visual cues present in a waveform display with one of the earliest works being Chiba & Kajiyama (1941). The best work comes from Scott (1980). Scott's work described regular patterns within the pitch periods of vowels, but was unable to assess how those patterns categorize and distinguish the vowel space. Since Scott's work, there is limited work with speech waveforms despite the advances in other fields derived from waveform analysis (Burke-Hubbard, 1998).

There are a number of competing models of speech perception (see Klatt, 1988), none of which can account for all of the following: (1) extracting formant frequencies and reconstructing vocal tract shapes; (2) accounting for variability, especially cross-speaker variability; and (3) accounting for temporal variability. The Waveform

Model can account for all these factors as well as explain perceptual errors for vowels.

The work by Peterson and Barney (1952) reported average formant values, which were used to create the initial parameters of the Waveform Model. As the specific values of pitch and the formants from 20 talkers were recorded and analyzed in the experiments described below, the categorical boundaries and error predictions became more refined and specific. The specific values allowed for the parameters to be much more detailed than averages could achieve. To simplify and limit the explanation of the model, the initial discussion will be limited to male speakers. Discussion of female talkers will follow Experiment II described below.

The lowest frequency in a complex waveform is the fundamental frequency (F0). Formants are frequency regions of relatively great intensity in the sound spectrum of a vowel, with F1 referring to the first formant, F2 referring to the second formant, and so on. From the average F0 (average pitch) and F1 values reported by Peterson and Barney (1952), a vowel can be categorized into one of six main categories by virtue of the interactions between F1 and F0. The relative categorical boundaries are established by the number of F1 cycles per pitch period, with the following rules determining how a vowel is first assigned to a main vowel category.

Category 1: $1 <$ F1 cycles per F0 < 2
Category 2: $2 <$ F1 cycles per F0 < 3
Category 3: $3 <$ F1 cycles per F0 < 4
Category 4: $4 <$ F1 cycles per F0 < 5
Category 5: $5.0 <$ F1 cycles per F0 < 5.5
Category 6: $5.5 <$ F1 cycles per F0 < 6.0

Each main category consists of a vowel pair, with the exception of Categories 3 and 6, which have only one vowel. Once a vowel waveform has been assigned to one of these categories, identification is reduced to making a further distinction between the vowel pairs.

One vowel within each categorical pair (Categories 1, 2, 4, and 5) has a third acoustic wave present (visually), while the other vowel of the pair does not. The presence of F2 in the range of 2000 Hz can be recognized visually as this third wave, but F2 values in the range of 1000 Hz have no visually discernable features. Since each main category has one vowel with F2 in the range of 2000 Hz and one vowel in the range of 1000 Hz (see Table 1), F2 frequencies provide an easily distinguished feature between the categorical vowel pairs. In fact, this is directly analogous to the distinguishing feature between the stop consonants /b/-/p/, /d/-/t/, and /g/-/k/ (the presence or absence of voicing). F2 values in the range of 2000 Hz are analogous to voicing being added to /b/, /d/, and /g/, while F2 values in the range of 1000 Hz are analogous to the voiceless quality of the consonants /p/, /t/, and /k/. Considering this similarity with an established pattern of phoneme perception, the model of vowel perception described here appears more than plausible.

Table 1 - *Waveform Model Organization of the Vowel Space*
Formants values from Peterson, G.E., & Barney, H.L. (1952).

Vowel - Category	F0	F1	F2	F3	F1-FO/100	F1/FO
/i/ - 1	136	270	2290	3010	1.35	1.99
/u/ - 1	141	300	870	2240	1.59	2.13
/I/ - 2	135	390	1990	2550	2.55	2.89
/U/ - 2	137	440	1020	2240	3.03	3.21
/er/ - 3	133	490	1350	1690	3.57	3.68
/ ɛ / - 4	130	530	1840	2480	4.00	4.08
/ɔ/ - 4	129	570	840	2410	4.41	4.42
/æ/ - 5	130	660	1720	2410	5.30	5.08
/ʌ/ - 5	127	640	1190	2390	5.13	5.04
/a/ - 6	124	730	1090	2440	6.06	5.89

Identification of the vowel /er/ (the lone member of Category 3) is also aided by the presence of a third acoustic wave. However, the appearance of this wave for this vowel does not conform to the categorical pair's appearance. This particular third wave is unique and provides additional information that distinguishes /er/ from neighboring categorical pairs. The vowel /a/ (the lone member of Category 6), follows the format of Categories 1, 2, 4, and 5, but it does not have a high F2 vowel paired with it, possibly due to articulatory limitations.

A successful model of vowel perception should also be able to explain other relationships associated with vowels. As mentioned above, the categorized vowel space described here is analogous to the stop consonants /b/-/p/, /d/-/t/, and /g/-/k/. To extend the analogy and the similarities, each categorical vowel pair should share a common articulatory gesture that establishes the categorical boundaries. In other words, each vowel within a category should share an articulatory gesture that produces a similar F1 value since it is F1 that varies between categories (F0 remains relatively constant). Furthermore, there should be an articulatory difference between categorical pairs that produces the difference in F2 frequencies, similar to the addition of voicing or not by vibrating the vocal folds. The following section organizes the articulatory gestures involved in vowel production by the six main categories.

From Table 2, it can be seen that the common articulatory gesture between categorical pairs is tongue height. Each categorical pair shares the same height of the tongue in the oral cavity, meaning the air flow through the oral cavity is being unobstructed at the same height within a category. This appears to be the common place of articulation for each category as /b/-/p/, /d/-/t/, and /g/-/k/ share a common place of articulation. It should also be noted that the tongue position provides an articulatory difference within each category by alternating the portion of the tongue that is lowered to open the airflow through the oral cavity. One vowel within a category has the airflow altered at the front of the oral cavity, while the other vowel in a category has the airflow altered at the back. The subtle difference in the unobstructed length of the oral cavity determined by where the airflow is altered by the tongue (front or back) is the likely source of the 30 to 50 cps difference between vowels of the same category. Although this is probably a valuable cue for the auditory system when identifying a vowel, this difference provides little information when visually identifying a vowel from the raw complex waveform. Fortunately, there is a visual cue that can distinguish between categorical pairs.

Table 2 - *Articulatory relationships*
Articulatory positions from Ladefoged, P. (1982).

Vowel - Category	Relative Tongue Positions	F1	Relative Lip Position	F2
/i/ - 1	high, front	270	unrounded, spread	2290
/u/ - 1	high, back	300	rounded	870
/I/ - 2	mid-high, front	390	unrounded, spread	1990
/U/ - 2	mid-high, back	440	rounded	1020
/er/ - 3	rhotacization	490	retroflex	1350 (F3=1690)
/ ɛ / - 4	mid, front	530	unrounded	1840
/ɔ/ - 4	mid, back	570	rounded	840
/æ/ - 5	low, front	660	unrounded	1720
/ʌ/ - 5	mid-low, back	640	rounded	1190
/a/ - 6	low, back	730	rounded	1090

As mentioned above, there is a third wave (high frequency, low amplitude) present in one of the categorical vowel pairs which visually distinguishes it from the other vowel in the category. From Table 3, one sees that one vowel from each pair is produced with the lips rounded, and the other vowel is produced with the lips spread or unrounded. An F2 in the range of 2000 Hz clearly appears to be associated with having the lips spread or unrounded. Therefore, having the lips spread or unrounded is directly analogous to vibrating the vocal folds during the production of /b/, /d/, and /g/ to add the voicing that distinguishes them from /p/, /t/, and /k/, respectively. Furthermore, rounding the lips (resulting in an F2 in the range of 1000 Hz) during vowel production is analogous to the voiceless quality of /p/, /t/, and /k/.

By organizing the vowel space in this way, it is possible to predict perceptual errors. The confusion data shown in Table 3 has Categories 1, 2, 4, and 5 organized in that order. Category 3 (/er/) is not in Table 3 because its formant values (placing it in the "middle" of the vowel space) make it a unique case to explain. Specifically, the distinct F2 and F3 values of /er/ necessitate an extension to the general rule described below. Rather than distract from the general rule explaining confusions between the four categorical pairs, the acoustic boundaries and errors involving /er/ will be discussed in the experimental evidence below. Furthermore, even though /a/ follows the general format of error prediction described below, Category 6 is not shown since /a/ does not have a categorical mate and many dialects have difficulty differentiating between /a/ and / ɔ /.

The Waveform Model predicts that errors occur across category boundaries, but only similar F2 vowels are confused for each other. In other words, a vowel with an F2 in the range of 2000 Hz will be confused for another vowel with an F2 in the range of 2000 Hz. Similarly, this is the case for vowels with F2 in the range of 1000 Hz. Vowel confusions are the result of misperceiving the number of F1 cycles per pitch period. In this way, F2 frequencies limit the number of possibilities as error candidates. Also as expected, confusions are more likely with a near neighbor (separated by one F1 cycle per pitch period) than with a distant neighbor (separated by two or more F1 cycles per pitch period). From the four categories that are shown, 2,983 out of 3,025 errors (98.61%) can be explained by searching for neighboring vowels with similar F2 frequencies.

Table 3 - *Error Prediction*
Error data reported by Peterson, G.E., and Barney, H.L. (1952).

Vowels Intended by Speaker	Vowels as Classified by Listeners							
	/i/-/u/		/I/ - /U/		/ɛ/ - /ɔ/		/æ/ - /ʌ/	
/i/	10,267 -		4	---	6	3	---	---
/u/		- 10,196	---	78	1	---	---	---
/I/	6	---	9,549	---	694	1	2	---
/U/	---	96	---	9,924	1	51	1	171
/ɛ/	---	---	257	---	9,014	3	949	2
/ɔ/	---	5	---	71	1	9,534	2	62
/æ/	---	---	1	---	300	2	9,919	15
/ʌ/	---	---	1	103	1	127	8	9,476

To this point, the vowel /er/ in Category 3 has not been discussed in detail. It is convenient for the waveform model that the one vowel that has a unique lip articulatory style when compared to the other vowels of the vowel space results in formant values that lie between the formant values of neighboring categories. This is especially evident when the F2 and F3 values of /er/ are compared to the other categories. Both the F2 and F3 values lie between the ranges of 1000 Hz to 2000 Hz of the other categories. With the lips already being directly associated with F2 values, the unique retroflex position of the lips to produce /er/ further demonstrates the role of the lips in F2 values, as well as F3 in the case of /er/. The quality of a unique lip position during vowel production produces a unique F2 and F3 value.

The first demonstration of the ability to identify vowels from visual displays of waveforms was presented in 1996 (Stokes, 1996). In that experiment, waveform displays of nine vowel productions from two Midwestern males were presented for identification. For each talker, subject MAS was presented with the nine waveforms of the speakers in random order by an experimenter. The subject was allowed to review each waveform before a final response was given and scored. The results showed that subject MAS correctly identified 5 out of 9 vowels for both speakers. The 55% accuracy across the vowel space of two speakers was well above chance (chance would be 1 correct out of 9 vowels per talker) and demonstrated the potential success of the model and how the cues are unaffected by talker variability. The 1996 study was replicated and extended to a female talker in 2001 (Stokes, 2001). In that study, subject MAS successfully identified 4 out of 9 vowels and 6 out of 9 vowels for two additional male speakers (again, 55% accuracy across these two talkers) and 4 out of 9 vowels for a female speaker (44% accuracy).

Despite the success of the two visual identification experiments, the method was subjective and difficult to replicate. The present study eliminates the subjectivity and provides a method that can easily be replicated. The analysis of the results also served to refine the categorical and distinguishing feature boundaries.

CHAPTER 2

EXPERIMENT I

Method

Subjects

A talker database of h-vowel-d (hVd) productions (Mullennix, 1994) was used as the source of vowels analyzed for this study. The entire database consists of 33 male and 44 female college students in Detroit, MI, who produced three tokens for each of the ten American English vowels. The recordings were made using CSRE software (Jamieson et al., 1992) and converted to .wav files using the TFR software package (Avaaz Innovations Inc., 1998). Of the 33 male talkers in the database, 20 were randomly selected for use in the current experiment. In the original experiments demonstrating identification of vowels by visual inspection of the waveforms (Stokes, 1996 and 2001), five talkers from the talker database (4 males and 1 female) were used. None of the unique talkers used in those experiments were used in the experiments presented here.

Apparatus

The nine vowels used in this study were / i /, / u /, / I /, / U /, / er /, / ε /, / $\jmath$ /, / æ /, / ^ /. Although the vowel /a/ is available in the database, it was excluded from this study since many Midwestern dialects have difficulty differentiating between /a/ and / $\jmath$ /. In most cases, there were three productions for each of the nine vowels used (27 productions per talker), but there were instances of only two productions for a given vowel by a talker. Across the 20 talkers, there were 524 vowels analyzed and every vowel was produced at least twice by each talker.

The research was performed on a Compaq Presario 2100 laptop computer, and the speech signal processing was performed with the TFR software. The collected data was entered into a Microsoft Access database where the data was mined and queried using the SQL query language. The programming language Cold Fusion was used to display the data and results in a browser. Within the Cold Fusion program, the necessary calculations and the conditional if-then logic were programmed. This allowed for quick modifications to the model parameters used to categorize and identify the vowel space. As errors occurred, modifications to the values used in the conditional logic (for example, the defined range of F2 values) for a vowel could be edited to eliminate the error. The programming and query languages made the error reduction process quick, and provided various statistics such as processing time.

Design
The speech signal processing begins by identifying the center of each vowel (within 10 ms) in order to make the pitch and formant frequency measurements at the most neutral and stable portion of the vowel. Figure 1 shows the display of the production of "whod" by Talker 12. From this display, the cursor can be placed in the relative center of the vowel to identify the time within the display associated with the center. A range of between 20 and 30 ms of that point in time can be used as the point in time that the pitch and formant values will be measured.

Once the relative center of the vowel is identified, the fundamental frequency was measured first so that the specific time that the measurements were made was not associated with an unusually high or low pitch frequency compared to the rest of the central portion of the vowel. The Cepstrum method (i.e., taking the Fourier Transform of the decibel spectrum) within TFR was used to perform the pitch extraction. Figure 2 shows the Cepstrum display for the "whod" production by Talker 12. Using the time identified from the display in Figure 1, the pitch measurement can be made at this central point in time. The point in time and the F0 value were recorded before performing the formant analysis.

The F1, F2, and F3 frequency measurements were made at the same point in time as the pitch measurement using the Formant Module in TFR. Figure 3 shows the Formant Module display of the production of "whod" by Talker 12 which is a typical visual display used during the formant measurement process. These measurements were recorded with the time and pitch from the display in Figure 2 before moving to the next vowel to be analyzed. For each production, the intended vowels identity, the point in time for the measurements, and the F0, F1, F2, and F3 values were recorded and entered into the Access database to be used in the computer recognition perceptual experiment.

Figure 1

This is a display of the entire vowel file to identify the relative center of the vowel.

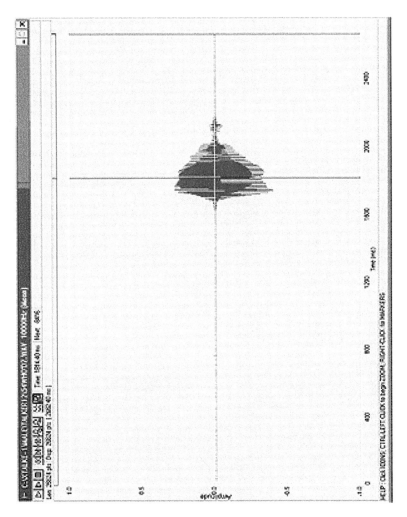

Figure 2

This is a Cepstral pitch display used to measure F0 for the vowel.

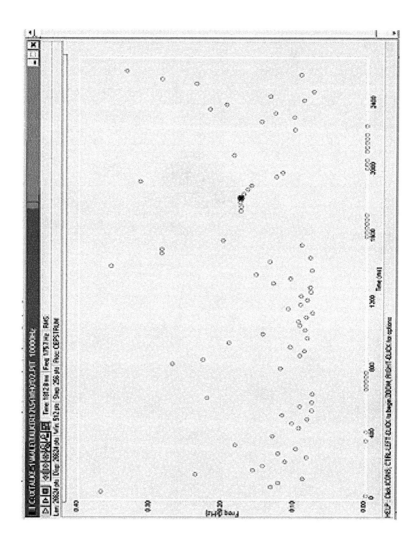

Figure 3

Formant display used to measure F1, F2, and F3 (without color).

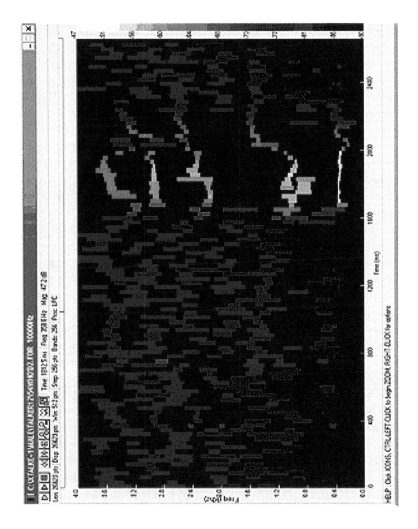

Procedure

To test the concepts in the model, the value of F1-F0/100 was used initially to calculate the number of F1 cycles per pitch period, and the F1, F2 and F3 values were retrieved for each vowel. By using conditional if-then logic, the model's parameters were used to identify the vowels. Specifically, the F1 to F0 ratio, and the F1, F2, and F3 values could be used in the conditional statements within the computer program. If the values of a vowel meet the conditional ranges, that vowel was identified (correct or wrong) without going through the rest of the vowels yet to be processed after the vowel that was identified (processing occurs sequentially and would end once an identification was made). The model's vowel identification was then compared to the intended value of the production by the talker to measure accuracy. At this point, the process was completed for the vowel. Subsequent vowels were then processed using the same method until all 524 vowels were looped through and identified. Execution times ranged from 280 ms to 1.3 seconds to process and display the results of all 524 vowels.

The order of the talkers and vowels was random and did not affect the results when the order was changed. However, the order of the parameters used does affect the results. If the boundaries are too broad or overlap, the first set of conditions met becomes the perceptual identity of the model. This forces the model to be as detailed as possible and with as little overlap as possible of the categorical boundary parameters so a vowel is not identified prematurely. As time progressed, more data and refinements to the model parameters reduced the need for overlap of parameters so the order of processing was not a factor.

As more talkers were analyzed, more data was available to refine the boundaries between vowels and go well beyond the averages documented by Peterson and Barney (1952) which were used to develop the initial parameters of the model. The final detailed boundaries between vowels are the result of analysis of the errors generated in the early trials. The elimination of the errors by adjusting the categorical boundaries was used to refine the boundaries to achieve the highest percent of accuracy across the 20 talkers. The specific boundaries and order of the conditions will be discussed in more detail below.

Results

Table 4 - *Vowel Identification Results Across Talkers*

Talker	Total Vowels	Total Correct	Percent Correct
1	27	26	96.30
2	26	26	100.00
3	23	22	95.65
4	27	26	96.30
5	27	25	92.59
6	27	27	100.00
7	27	25	92.59
8	26	23	88.46
9	27	26	96.30
10	27	25	92.59
12	27	27	100.00
13	26	25	96.15
15	25	22	88.00
16	26	21	80.77
17	27	24	88.89
18	27	26	96.30
19	26	26	100.00
20	26	26	100.00
22	26	22	84.62
26	24	22	91.67
Totals	524	492	93.89

Table 4 shows the percent correct vowel identification across talkers. Five talkers were identified perfectly, five talkers were identified at a 96% correct rate or better, and five talkers had a percent correct between 96% and 91% with 14 out of 20 talkers being identified over 92.5% correct or better. Three talkers fell between 88% and 91% correct, and two talkers fell between 85% and 80% correct. It should be noted that two talkers (talkers #11 and #14) were not used in this experiment due to a unique quality to their productions. However, they will be discussed again in Chapter 4 (Exceptions and a Female Talker). It is expected that detailed analysis of these talkers will provide additional cues to be incorporated into the Waveform Model. For the 20 talkers that were used in this experiment, the waveform model correctly identified 492 of the 524 vowels for an overall 93.9% correct identification.

Table 5 - *Vowel Identification Results Across Vowels*

Vowel	Total Vowels	Total Correct	Percent Correct
heed	60	60	100.00
whod	58	57	98.28
hid	59	59	100.00
hood	59	58	98.31
heard	58	58	100.00
had	57	43	75.44
head	57	49	85.96
hawed	56	52	92.86
hud	60	56	93.33
Totals	524	492	93.89

Table 5 shows that 3 of the 9 vowels used in the study were identified perfectly, two vowels were identified at 98% or better, two vowels fell between 92% and 94%, and two vowels fell between 75% and 86% correct. Of the 32 total errors, almost half were associated with / æ / productions which accounted for 14 errors and 43.7% of the total number of errors. Another 8 errors (25% of the total) are associated with / ɛ /, and combined these two vowels accounted for 69% of the total errors. Because the program logic is set so the first vowel that meets the criteria is selected as the vowel, "head" productions would account for 14 errors if the order of the parameters for each vowel was reversed. For this experiment, the confusion between "head" and "had" was the greatest source of errors which is further illustrated in Table 6.

Table 6 - *Experiment I Confusion Data*

Vowels Intended by Speaker	Vowels as Classified by the Waveform Model							
	/i/-	/u/	/I/ -	/U/	/ ɛ / -	/ ɔ/	/æ/ -	/ʌ/
/i/	60	---	---	---	---	---	---	---
/u/	---	57	---	*1*	---	---	---	---
/I/	---	---	59	---	---	---	---	---
/U/	---	---	---	58	---	---	---	*1*
/ ɛ /	---	---	*2*	---	49	---	*6*	---
/ɔ/	---	---	---	---	---	52	---	*4*
/æ/	---	---	*2*	---	*12*	---	43	---
/ʌ/	---	---	---	*1*	---	*3*	---	56

Table 6 shows the confusion data resulting from the model's performance. The concept that errors will occur for categorical neighboring vowels with a similar F2 frequency is demonstrated in these results. All 32 errors occurred between neighboring vowels with high frequency F2 vowels being confused for other high frequency F2 vowels, and low frequency F2 vowels being confused with each other. Table 6 shows that in addition to the 93.9% overall accuracy across 20 talkers, 100% of the errors was fully explainable by examining the architecture of the model.

Further analysis has led to a more refined categorical classification for the vowel space when compared to the values displayed in Table 1. Using actual data points compared to averages allowed for refinement of the parameters. As each new talker was analyzed the parameters could be expanded to correctly identify each new talker added to the database. Setting the parameters to correctly identify 100% of the utterances from one individual talker was relatively easy using the models basic principles, but the ultimate goal was to achieve that level of accuracy for all talkers. As new talker measurements were added to the database, analysis was performed on the misperceptions, the ratio values, and formant values. Eventually this led to the 93.9% overall accuracy in this experiment. To this point, this was the best that could be achieved with the parameters and calculations discussed here.

The parameters displayed in Table 7 are the values achieving the highest level of accuracy across all 20 talkers in the present experiment. This does not mean that further modifications cannot be made to these parameters to improve performance, but from the original starting point derived from the average values reported by Peterson and Barney (1952) this was a significant refinement of the parameters. The individual F1 values may play a role in vowel identification and could be used to refine the parameters, but it was not obvious at the time of this experiment what that role may be. Several modifications were made to the parameter values and the order of the parameter processing, but the sequence and range of values achieving the highest accuracy are represented here. Changing the sequence does have an effect, but it is limited because there is not a great deal of overlap across boundaries. Although this configuration of parameters produced the best results, other variations were intriguing and may be worth pursuing at some point.

Table 7 - *Experiment I: Waveform Model Parameters Based on Perceptual Results*

Vowel	F1-F0/100 (as R)	F2	F3
/ i / - heed	R < 2.4	1400 < F2	1800 < F3
/ u / - whod	R < 2.835	F2 < 1400	1800 < F3
/ I / - hid	2.4 < R < 3.685	1550 < F2	1950 < F3
/ I / - hid	3.685 < R < 4.08	1904 < F2	1950 < F3
/ U / - hood	2.835 < R < 4.3	1550 < F2	1950 < F3
/ er / - heard	2.3 < R < 4.65	1150 < F2 < 1650	F3 < 1950
/ ɛ / - head	3.685 < R < 4.08	1550 < F2 < 1904	1950 < F3
/ ɛ / - head	4.08 < R < 4.3	1550 < F2 < 1936	1950 < F3
/ ɛ / - head	4.3 < R < 6.15	1447 < F2 < 1838.2	1950 < F3
/ æ / - had	3.685 < R < 4.08	1904 < F2	1950 < F3
/ æ / - had	4.08 < R < 4.3	1936 < F2	1950 < F3
/ æ / - had	4.3 < R < 6.15	1838.2 < F2	1950 < F3
/ ^ / - hud	4.3 < R < 5.0	F2 < 1447	1950 < F3
/ ^ / - hud	5.0 < R < 5.97	1123 < F2 < 1447	1950 < F3
/ ɔ / - hawed	5.0 < R < 5.97	F2 < 1123	1950 < F3
/ ɔ / - hawed	5.97 < R < 7.2	F2 < 1387	1950 < F3

CHAPTER 3

EXPERIMENT II

This experiment calculated the relationship of F1 to F0 differently than Experiment I, but the underlying foundation of the waveform model was maintained. A vowel was categorized using the ratio of F1 to F0, and then a vowel was distinguished from the categorical pair with a relatively high or low F2 value.

Method

Subjects/ Apparatus/ Design

The subjects, apparatus, and design are exactly the same as in Experiment I. The primary difference between Experiment I and II was the method of calculating the relationship of F1 to F0. The consequences of this methodological change will be described below.

Procedure

F1-F0/100 was used in Experiment I to calculate the number of F1 cycles per pitch period. The ratio F1/F0 does not generate dramatically different values compared to the F1–F0/100 values (see table 1), but any change to the F1 to F0 ratio is significant since the initial condition and categorization element of the Waveform Model is F1 to F0. Modifying the program to reflect this method change involved modifying the one line in the program used to calculate the F1 to F0 ratio.

Beyond the F1/F0 ratio calculation, the F1, F2, and F3 values are also available as parameters that can be utilized for identification. Although F3 was only used to distinguish /er/ productions and F1 was not used beyond the calculation of F1-F0/100, there were indications that F1 and F3 had the potential for playing a larger role in the identification process. Table 8 shows the final parameters used in Experiment II. The method of analyzing the errors to edit the values of the categorical boundaries and distinguishing cues used in this experiment is the same as Experiment I.

Table 8 - *Experiment II: Waveform Model Parameters from Perceptual Results*

Vowel	F1/F0 (as R)	F1	F2	F3
/ er / - heard	1.8 < R < 4.65		1150 < F2 < 1650	F3 < 1950
/ i / - heed	R < 2.0		2090 < F2	1950 < F3
/ i / - heed	R < 3.1	276 < F1 < 385	2090 < F2	1950 < F3
/ u / - whod	3.0 < R < 3.1	F1 < 406	F2 < 1200	1950 < F3
/ u / - whod	R < 3.05	290 < F1 < 434	F2 < 1360	1800 < F3
/ I / - hid	2.2 < R < 3.0	385 < F1 < 620	1667 < F2 < 2293	1950 < F3
/ U / - hood	2.3 < R < 2.97	433 < F1 < 563	1039 < F2 < 1466	1950 < F3
/ æ / - had	2.4 < R < 3.14	540 < F1 < 626	2015 < F2 < 2129	1950 < F3
/ I / - hid	3.0 < R < 3.5	417 < F1 < 503	1837 < F2 < 2119	1950 < F3
/ U / - hood	2.98 < R < 3.4	415 < F1 < 734	1017 < F2 < 1478	1950 < F3
/ ɛ / - head	3.01 < R < 3.41	541 < F1 < 588	1593 < F2 < 1936	1950 < F3
/ æ / - had	3.14 < R < 3.4	540 < F1 < 654	1940 < F2 < 2129	1950 < F3
/ I / - hid	3.5 < R < 3.97	462 < F1 < 525	1841 < F2 < 2061	1950 < F3
/ U / - hood	3.5 < R < 4.0	437 < F1 < 551	1078 < F2 < 1502	1950 < F3

Vowel	F1/F0 (as R)	F1	F2	F3
/ ^ / - hud	3.5 < R < 3.99	562 < F1 < 787	1131 < F2 < 1313	1950 < F3
/ ɔ / - hawed	3.5 < R < 3.99	651 < F1 < 690	887 < F2 < 1023	1950 < F3
/ æ / - had	3.5 < R < 3.99	528 < F1 < 696	1875 < F2 < 2129	1950 < F3
/ ɛ / - head	3.5 < R < 3.99	537 < F1 < 702	1594 < F2 < 2144	1950 < F3
/ I / - hid	4.0 < R < 4.3	457 < F1 < 523	1904 < F2 < 2295	1950 < F3
/ U / - hood	4.0 < R < 4.3	475 < F1 < 560	1089 < F2 < 1393	1950 < F3
/ ^ / - hud	4.0 < R < 4.6	561 < F1 < 675	1044 < F2 < 1445	1950 < F3
/ ɔ / - hawed	4.0 < R < 4.67	651 < F1 < 749	909 < F2 < 1123	1950 < F3
/ æ / - had	4.0 < R < 4.6	592 < F1 < 708	1814 < F2 < 2095	1950 < F3
/ ɛ / - head	4.0 < R < 4.58	519 < F1 < 745	1520 < F2 < 1967	1950 < F3
/ ^ / - hud	4.62 < R < 5.01	602 < F1 < 705	1095 < F2 < 1440	1950 < F3
/ ɔ / - hawed	4.67 < R < 5.0	634 < F1 < 780	985 < F2 < 1176	1950 < F3
/ æ / - had	4.62 < R < 5.01	570 < F1 < 690	1779 < F2 < 1969	1950 < F3
/ ɛ /-head	4.59 < R < 4.95	596 < F1 < 692	1613 < F2 < 1838	1950 < F3
/ ɔ / - hawed	5.01 < R < 5.6	644 < F1 < 801	982 < F2 < 1229	1950 < F3

Vowel	F1/F0 (as R)	F1	F2	F3
/ ʌ / - hud	5.02 < R < 5.75	623 < F1 < 679	1102 < F2 < 1342	1950 < F3
/ ʌ / - hud	5.02 < R < 5.72	679 < F1 < 734	1102 < F2 < 1342	1950 < F3
/ æ / - had	5.0 < R < 5.5		1679 < F2 < 1807	1950 < F3
/ æ / - had	5.0 < R < 5.5		1844 < F2 < 1938	
/ ɛ / - head	5.0 < R < 5.5		1589 < F2 < 1811	
/ æ / - had	5.0 < R < 5.5		1842 < F2 < 2101	
/ ɔ / - hawed	5.5 < R < 5.95	680 < F1 < 828	992 < F2 < 1247	1950 < F3
/ ɛ / - head	5.5 < R < 6.1		1573 < F2 < 1839	
/ æ / - had	5.5 < R < 6.3		1989 < F2 < 2066	
/ ɛ / - head	5.5 < R < 6.3		1883 < F2 < 1989	2619 < F3
/ æ / - had	5.5. < R < 6.3		1839 < F2 < 1944	F3 < 2688
/ ɔ / - hawed	5.95 < R < 7.13	685 < F1 < 850	960 < F2 < 1267	1950 < F3

Note: Some cells do not have a value because it is not necessary to have the parameters beyond those listed to successfully identify a vowel without errors.

As the errors were analyzed, several things became apparent. First, the ratios were easier to comprehend and organize by having relatively smaller ranges for the boundaries. Ratio ranges of .5 or less were common in Experiment II, compared to ranges greater than .5

and over 1.0 that were prevalent in Experiment I. The smaller ranges means there are more conditional ranges to process compared to Experiment I, but this could be viewed as more detail being applied across the vowel space. Second, within these smaller ranges, vowels from other categories drift into what would be considered another categorical range. F2 values continue to distinguish the vowels within each of these ranges, but additional cues can be used to refine the category and make the F2 information more distinct in a smaller range. Third, F1 became a valuable cue to distinguish between the crowded ranges in the middle of the vowel space. As vowels drift into neighboring categorical ranges, F1 values aid in the categorization of the vowel since the F1 values appear to maintain a certain range for a given category regardless of the individuals pitch. Fourth, F3 values may have a role in distinguishing "head" and "had" and were used in a limited way in Experiment II. Overall, analysis of the data resulting from the use of F1/F0 led to the refined ranges and greater use of available cues to achieve the highest level of accuracy possible. The use of additional cues such as F1 was not obvious in Experiment I, but additional review of this cue is warranted. The final parameters used and the sequence of processing for Experiment II are shown in Table 8.

Results

Table 9 shows the percent correct vowel identification across talkers for Experiment II. Several significant improvements from the parameters used in this experiment can be seen including an overall 97.7% correct rate compared to 93.9% achieved in Experiment I. Furthermore, 100% correct identification was achieved for 12 of the 20 talkers which more than doubles the 100% correct observed for five talkers in Experiment I. The other eight talkers were correctly identified over 92% of the time with 4 of those 8 being identified at 96% or better. In Experiment I, six talkers were identified at a rate less than 92% which again reflects the improvements from the changes to the parameters used in Experiment II. This level of improvement across talkers is encouraging in that additional adjustments will lead toward perfect performance.

Table 9 - *Experiment II - Vowel Identification Results Across Talkers*

Talker	Total Vowels	Total Correct	Percent Correct
1	27	27	100
2	26	25	96.2
3	23	23	100
4	27	27	100
5	27	27	100
6	27	27	100
7	27	26	96.3
8	26	24	92.3
9	27	27	100
10	27	27	100
12	27	27	100
13	26	26	100
15	25	24	96
16	26	24	92.3
17	27	25	92.6
18	27	27	100
19	26	24	92.3
20	26	26	100
22	26	25	96.2
26	24	24	100
Totals	524	512	97.7

Table 10 shows the percent correct across vowels. Compared to the results from Experiment I, performance for each vowel stayed at 100% or improved. Of the nine vowels tested, five vowels were identified at 100% and 2 of the other 4 were identified over 98%. The other two vowels were at 87.7% and 95%. The largest source of errors is "head" with 7 of the 12 total errors being associated with "head". The confusions between "head" and "had" are closely related with the errors being reversed when the order of the parameters is reversed. Additional refinement is still needed to eliminate any overlap which would cause this reversal of errors and errors in general, but any refinement work will likely be focused on the relationship between "head" and "had".

Table 10 - *Experiment II - Vowel Identification Results Across Vowels*

Vowel	Total Vowels	Total Correct	Percent Correct
heed	60	60	100
whod	58	58	100
hid	59	59	100
hood	59	59	100
heard	58	58	100
had	57	56	98.2
head	57	50	87.7
hawed	56	55	98.2
hud	60	57	95
Totals	524	512	97.7

Table 11 shows the confusion data and further illustrates the head/had relationship. Beyond that, Table 11 also shows that 100% of the errors are accounted for by neighboring vowels, with vowels confused for other vowels across categories when they possess similar F2 values. This is a consistent result across both Experiment I and Experiment II.

Table 11 - *Experiment II Confusion Data*

Vowels Intended by Speaker	Vowels as Classified by the Waveform Model							
	/i/ - /u/		/I/-/U/		/ ɛ / - /ɔ/		/æ/ - /ʌ/	
/i/	60	---	---	---	---	---	---	---
/u/	---	58	---	---	---	---	---	---
/I/	---	---	59	---	---	---	---	---
/U/	---	---	---	59	---	---	---	---
/ ɛ /	---	---	*1*	---	50	---	*6*	---
/ɔ/	---	---	---	---	---	55	---	*1*
/æ/	---	---	---	---	*1*	---	56	---
/ʌ/	---	---	---	*1*	---	*2*	---	57

Table 8 shows the parameters with the highest level of accuracy. As mentioned above, there are more ranges because they span a smaller range of F1/F0 ratio values than in Experiment I. These ranges have multiple vowels, but F2 continues to be the main distinguishing cue within these ranges. As the number of vowels within a categorical range grew to as many as the six vowels within the F1/F0 ratio range of 3.5 – 4.0, F1 became a cue to refine and complete categorical membership. The F1/F0 ratio is flexible enough to account for talker variations regarding F0, and the ratios of vowels can cross a variety of boundaries. F1 refines the specific category for the vowel which maintains the role the F2 value plays in distinguishing between categorical pairs. F2 values distinguish a vowel after it has been properly categorized from the broad F1/F0 ratios and the specific F1 values.

A final point regarding Table 8 is the potential use of F3 as a distinguishing cue to differentiate vowels. Although F3 is currently being used for / er / identification and in the high F1/F0 ratio ranges, it showed potential as a distinguishing cue in the lower F1/F0 ratios. Several attempts were made to introduce F3 as a more prominent cue, but the F3 values were not consistent enough to be used.

However, several attempts were promising and analysis showed that F3 values may play a role on the categorical boundary edges and distinguishing between /head/ and /had/. Additional analysis may show how to use this cue more effectively, but categorizing a vowel with F1/F0 and F1 values and then using F2 as the distinguishing cue within a category is enough information to achieve the 97.7% accuracy.

CHAPTER 4

TWO EXCEPTIONS AND ONE FEMALE

Experiment I
There were two male talkers (Talkers #11 and #14 in the database) that were not used in Experiment I or Experiment II because of what ultimately proved to be unique characteristics of their productions. Despite attempts to categorize the vowels from these talkers in Experiment I, correct identification could not be improved much above 50% for these talkers and attempts to modify the parameters to improve the performance for them was detrimental to vowel identification for the other talkers. Tables 12 and 13 show the Experiment I results for these two male talkers with the formant values and the ratio of F1 to F0 calculated from F1 – F0/100. Upon reflection, the component values of each vowel lead to an explanation for the errors and address an important issue regarding the parameters used in Experiment I.

Table 12 - *Male Talker 11*
Experiment I results which uses F1-F0/100 for the ratio value.

Ratio	Model Vowel	Vowel Text	F0 Value	F1 Value	F2 Value	F3 Value
3.997	head	had1	185.2	584.9	1893.5	2444
4.156	head	had2	200	615.6	1874.2	2402.8
4.059	hid	had3	188.7	594.6	1952.5	2495.5
5.011	hawed	hawed1	169.5	670.6	1110.2	2402.2
4.624	hud	hawed2	192.3	654.7	1228.7	2459.1
5.961	hud	hawed3	188.7	784.8	1175.8	2516.6
3.796	hid	head1	192.3	571.9	1961.9	2504.3
3.71	hid	head2	208.3	579.3	1989.2	2489.2
2.767	hid	head3	212.8	489.5	2025.3	2501.9
2.637	heard	heard1	192.3	456	1414.4	1814.3
2.391	heed	heard2	212.8	451.9	1432.4	1935.6
2.429	heard	heard3	222.2	465.1	1388.2	1718.9

Ratio	Model Vowel	Vowel Text	F0 Value	F1 Value	F2 Value	F3 Value
1.582	heed	heed1	181.8	340	2377	2884.6
0.651	heed	heed2	243.9	309	2268.2	2714.4
0.475	heed	heed3	256.4	303.9	2338.8	2584.3
2.309	heed	hid1	217.4	448.3	2228.1	2627.4
2.616	hid	hid2	238.1	499.7	2383	2712.2
2.673	hid	hid3	256.4	523.7	2090.4	2599.3
2.341	whod	hood1	227.3	461.4	1377.9	2501.2
2.316	whod	hood2	232.6	464.2	1393.6	2347.2
2.54	whod	hood3	243.9	497.9	1267.2	2448.7
4.118	hood	hud1	204.1	615.9	1438.4	2599.1
4.086	hood	hud2	188.7	597.3	1479.6	2590.1
4.446	hud	hud3	227.3	671.9	1363	2519.5
0.791	whod	whod1	256.4	335.5	1049.1	2305
2.022	whod	whod2	238.1	440.3	970.2	2263.4
0.989	whod	whod3	243.9	342.8	1015.8	2314.2
12/27	0.444					

Table 13 - *Male Talker 14*
Experiment I results which uses F1-F0/100 for the ratio value.

Ratio	Model Vowel	Vowel Text	F0 Value	F1 Value	F2 Value	F3 Value
5.965	had	had1	151.5	748	1838.4	2549.9
7.048	no match	had2	212.8	917.6	1901.1	2588
5.931	head	had3	196.1	789.2	1794.1	2671.7
6.424	hawed	hawed1	192.3	834.7	1162.3	2831.8
6.841	hawed	hawed3	222.2	906.3	1146.5	2717.6
5.558	head	head1	147.1	702.9	1676.8	2540.9
5.499	head	head2	192.3	742.2	1683.8	2642.8
6.549	no match	head3	222.2	877.1	1727.1	2599.8
3.004	heard	heard1	285.7	586.1	1260.5	1670
2.613	heard	heard2	256.4	517.7	1250.5	1732.8
2.818	heard	heard3	277.8	559.6	1381.2	1671.5
2.063	heed	heed1	222.2	428.5	2398.7	2861.8

Ratio	Model Vowel	Vowel Text	F0 Value	F1 Value	F2 Value	F3 Value
1.549	heed	heed2	256.4	411.3	2398.9	2966.3
2.261	heed	heed3	250	476.1	2479.9	3176.5
4.911	had	hid2	238.1	729.2	1877	2581.4
2.593	hid	hid3	222.2	481.5	1936.1	2609.5
4.475	hud	hood1	222.2	669.7	1103.9	2836.4
5.818	hawed	hood2	263.2	845	1063.4	2641.9
2.701	whod	hood3	270.3	540.4	1070.4	2583.3
4.307	hud	hud1	212.8	643.5	1000.2	2736.4
4.248	hood	hud2	238.1	662.9	1124.5	2655.9
4.288	hood	hud3	227.3	656.1	1107.8	2783.5
2.325	whod	whod1	238.1	470.6	954.1	2390.8
2.21	whod	whod2	238.1	459.1	946.3	2387.9
2.624	whod	whod3	294.1	556.5	1029.7	2510.5
16 /25	0.64					

Use of the parameters in Experiment I resulted in 44% correct identification (12 out of 27) for Talker 11 and 64% correct (16 out of 25) for Talker 14. Beyond the large number of errors, there is one component of the vowels that was unique to these males. Typically, in terms of F0, male voices range from 100 Hz to 150 Hz, and female voices range from 170 Hz to 220 Hz. When examining these two male talkers, the average F0 across the vowel space for Talker 11 was 216 Hz and the average F0 for Talker 14 was 230 Hz. Thus, the average F0 for these two talkers averaged 223 Hz while the average F0 for the other 20 males used in Experiment I and II was 148 Hz. Since their F0 values were extremely high and outside the normal range for male voice (Peterson & Barney, 1952), this produced F1 to F0 ratios that were outside the boundaries of other male talkers (possessing lower F0 values) when using F1-F0/100. Thus, the F1–F0/100 ratio values fell outside the typical male categorical ranges, and one of the consequences was no identification for two of Talker 14's vowel productions. The parameters can be adjusted to correctly identify the two vowels the model did not identify (neither correct nor wrong), but this only would increase the accuracy for Talker 14 to 72% (18 out of 25 correct). More vowels that do not have a model match would be a better result since the parameters can be modified to correctly identify the vowel without generating a misperception for another talker. However, the limited number of no matches and the large number of misperceptions indicates a lack of flexibility across male talkers with a higher F0 than average.

To this point the male Talkers 11 and 14 are indicators of what a successful model will need to do to accommodate for higher frequency pitches like those produced by females and children. At least one female talker's productions needed to be analyzed and the measurements entered into the database to see if the parameters continue to have difficulty identifying vowels produced with an average F0 over 200 Hz. Table 14 shows the measurements of the first female analyzed and subjected to the model using Experimental I parameters. Her overall F0 average is 253 Hz, resulting in productions 37 Hz higher in pitch compared to Talker 11 and 23 Hz higher than Talker 14. These three talkers average between 68 and 105 Hz higher than the average of 148 Hz for the 20 males used in Experiments I and II.

Table 14 - *Female Talker 1*
Experiment I results which uses F1 - F0/100 for the ratio value.

Ratio	Model Vowel	Vowel Text	F0 Value	F1 Value	F2 Value	F3 Value
7.45	no match	had1	226.8	971.8	2217.3	2966.1
7.645	no match	had2	227.7	992.2	2396.2	2990.2
7.36	no match	had3	222.1	958.1	2118.5	2998.4
7.484	no match	hawed1	228.3	976.7	1237.5	2987.2
7.588	no match	hawed2	232.8	991.6	1267.6	2995.5
7.533	no match	hawed3	232.3	985.6	1259.2	2986.4
8.269	no match	head1	243.9	1070.8	2086.4	3090.6
7.292	no match	head2	212.9	942.1	2066	2979.6
7.848	no match	head3	232.9	1017.7	2014.1	3061.2
7.17	no match	heard1	263.6	980.6	1433.9	1983.2
7.57	no match	heard2	276.8	1033.8	1448.3	2022.8
6.495	no match	heard3	263	912.5	1401	1930.4
0.407	M-heed	heed1	303	343.7	1770.3	2750.1
0.764	M-heed	heed2	303	379.4	1593.3	2959.4
1.412	M-heed	heed3	294.1	435.3	1667.7	2939.1
6.574	no match	hid1	244.6	902	2196	3038.8
6.084	M-had	hid2	243.2	851.6	2349.6	3040.8

Ratio	Model Vowel	Vowel Text	F0 Value	F1 Value	F2 Value	F3 Value
6.13	M-had	hid3	232.3	845.3	2275.6	3006.9
3.241	M-hood	hood1	278.6	602.7	1202.4	2979.4
3.251	M-hood	hood2	278.6	603.7	1211.8	2996
5.609	M-hud	hud1	243.7	804.6	1327.8	2939.6
5.501	M-hud	hud2	243.7	793.8	1330.6	2976.3
5.391	M-head	hud3	237.6	776.7	1460.1	3009.1
3.979	M-hood	whod1	305.9	703.8	1308.2	2955
2.935	M-hood	whod3	262.4	555.9	1414.3	2805.7
7/25	0.28					

Although the performance in Table 14 shows 28% accuracy (7 out of 25 correct), over half (13) of the vowels were not identified by the parameters used in Experiment I. This means additional ranges could be added or the existing ranges could be modified to identify these vowels without affecting the accuracy of other talkers. This would increase the accuracy for this female to 80% (20 out of 25 correct) which would be better than the performance for Talkers 11 and 14. If a correct identification is not made, the desired result for any new talker added to the testing would be to have no model match in order to improve the ranges and parameter boundaries. Since no conditional statement matched a particular vowel, it is the equivalent of a future correct identification and the model's conditional logic is improved. The parameters do not encompass the values in the conditional logic, so the parameters can be expanded to create a correct identification without creating an error for another vowel. With so many vowels without a match, many parameters would be improved by accounting for these higher pitch vowels produced by Female Talker 1.

Accounting for the female productions without a match has the potential for improving the performance of Talkers 11 and 14. Since they all share a relatively high F0 compared to the other talkers used in these experiments, the adjustments to correctly identify one talker may correctly capture the other vowels sharing a relatively high pitch. However, the majority of the errors for Talkers 11 and 14 were confusions. This means these vowels share parameters with other vowels, which reflects a limitation of the model since overlap of categorical parameters should be as limited as possible to eliminate errors. As these higher pitch productions are analyzed and the parameters are improved to the point of highest performance, it would be hoped that the analysis of these enhancements will limit categorical boundary overlap and possibly improve performance for all the talkers measured up to this point.

Attempts have been made to account for these vowels, but no adjustments have resulted in better accuracy than what was achieved as shown in Tables 12 through 14. The model parameters used in Experiment I can be adjusted to correctly match the unidentified vowels, but this does not improve the performance for the other 20 talkers and the performance is still worse than the other 20 talkers and would bring down overall accuracy. Further analysis may yield alternative values to improve performance for the Experiment I parameters, but analysis of the higher frequency talkers using Experiment II parameters requires testing also.

Experiment II

Tables 15, 16, and 17 show the results for male talkers 11 and 14 and female talker 1 using the parameters of Experiment II. Beginning with Talker 11, only 33% correct was achieved (9 out of 27 correct), with 12 of the errors involving no match at all. These vowels can be identified through parameter modifications (without creating errors for other talkers) so the percent correct would go to 78% (21 out of 27 correct). Additional analysis would be needed to try and reconcile the remaining errors and little time has been spent on this talker within the Experiment II method at this time. Even though 78% is still below the 97.7% achieved in Experiment II, it is well above the 44% described above when tested with the Experiment I parameters. The Experiment II parameters appear to be flexible enough to account for the higher frequency of Talker 11 better than the methods used in Experiment I. More time is needed to analyze this unique talker in order to achieve a level of accuracy above 78%.

Talker 14 shows even more promise within the method of Experiment II. Of the 25 vowels, seven were correctly identified producing a 28% accuracy rate, but all 18 errors involved no model match. Once these are resolved, this would result in 100% correct. Experiment I achieved 72%, but again the method used in Experiment II proves flexible enough to accommodate a variety of pitches in a way the method used in Experiment I cannot. This is demonstrated by the limited effort needed to bring a new talker into the model with a unique pitch and achieve 100% accuracy for that talker.

Table 15 - *Male Talker 11*
Exp. II results using F1/F0 for the ratio value.

Ratio	Model Vowel	Vowel Text	F0 Value	F1 Value	F2 Value	F3 Value
3.158	head	had1	185.2	584.9	1893.5	2444
3.078	no match	had2	200	615.6	1874.2	2402.8
3.151	had	had3	188.7	594.6	1952.5	2495.5
3.956	no match	hawed1	169.5	670.6	1110.2	2402.2
3.405	no match	hawed2	192.3	654.7	1228.7	2459.1
4.159	no match	hawed3	188.7	784.8	1175.8	2516.6
2.974	Hid	head1	192.3	571.9	1961.9	2504.3
2.781	Hid	head2	208.3	579.3	1989.2	2489.2
2.3	Hid	head3	212.8	489.5	2025.3	2501.9
2.371	heard	heard1	192.3	456	1414.4	1814.3
2.124	heard	heard2	212.8	451.9	1432.4	1935.6
2.093	heard	heard3	222.2	465.1	1388.2	1718.9
1.87	heed	heed1	181.8	340	2377	2884.6
1.267	heed	heed2	243.9	309	2268.2	2714.4
1.185	heed	heed3	256.4	303.9	2338.8	2584.3
2.062	no match	hid1	217.4	448.3	2228.1	2627.4
2.099	no match	hid2	238.1	499.7	2383	2712.2
2.043	no match	hid3	256.4	523.7	2090.4	2599.3
2.03	no match	hood1	227.3	461.4	1377.9	2501.2
1.996	no match	hood2	232.6	464.2	1393.6	2347.2
2.041	no match	hood3	243.9	497.9	1267.2	2448.7
3.018	hood	hud1	204.1	615.9	1438.4	2599.1
3.165	no match	hud2	188.7	597.3	1479.6	2590.1
2.956	whod	hud3	227.3	671.9	1363	2519.5
1.309	whod	whod1	256.4	335.5	1049.1	2305
1.849	no match	whod2	238.1	440.3	970.2	2263.4
1.405	whod	whod3	243.9	342.8	1015.8	2314.2
9/27	0.333					

Table 16- *Male Talker 14*
Experiment II results which uses F1/F0 for the ratio value.

Ratio	Model Vowel	Vowel Text	F0 Value	F1 Value	F2 Value	F3 Value
4.937	no match	had1	151.5	748	1838.4	2549.9
4.312	no match	had2	212.8	917.6	1901.1	2588
4.025	no match	had3	196.1	789.2	1794.1	2671.7
4.341	no match	hawed1	192.3	834.7	1162.3	2831.8
4.078	no match	hawed3	222.2	906.3	1146.5	2717.6
4.778	no match	head1	147.1	702.9	1676.8	2540.9
3.86	no match	head2	192.3	742.2	1683.8	2642.8
3.947	no match	head3	222.2	877.1	1727.1	2599.8
2.051	heard	heard1	285.7	586.1	1260.5	1670
2.019	heard	heard2	256.4	517.7	1250.5	1732.8
2.014	heard	heard3	277.8	559.6	1381.2	1671.5
1.928	heed	heed1	222.2	428.5	2398.7	2861.8
1.604	heed	heed2	256.4	411.3	2398.9	2966.3
1.904	heed	heed3	250	476.1	2479.9	3176.5
3.063	no match	hid2	238.1	729.2	1877	2581.4
2.167	no match	hid3	222.2	481.5	1936.1	2609.5
3.014	hood	hood1	222.2	669.7	1103.9	2836.4
3.21	no match	hood2	263.2	845	1063.4	2641.9
1.999	no match	hood3	270.3	540.4	1070.4	2583.3
3.024	no match	hud1	212.8	643.5	1000.2	2736.4
2.784	no match	hud2	238.1	662.9	1124.5	2655.9
2.886	no match	hud3	227.3	656.1	1107.8	2783.5
1.976	no match	whod1	238.1	470.6	954.1	2390.8
1.928	no match	whod2	238.1	459.1	946.3	2387.9
1.892	no match	whod3	294.1	556.5	1029.7	2510.5
7/25	0.28					

Table 17 - *Female Talker 1*
Experiment II results which uses F1/F0 for the ratio value.

Ratio	Model Vowel	Vowel Text	F0 Value	F1 Value	F2 Value	F3 Value
4.285	no match	had1	226.8	971.8	2217.3	2966.1
4.357	no match	had2	227.7	992.2	2396.2	2990.2
4.314	no match	had3	222.1	958.1	2118.5	2998.4
4.278	no match	hawed1	228.3	976.7	1237.5	2987.2
4.259	no match	hawed2	232.8	991.6	1267.6	2995.5
4.243	no match	hawed3	232.3	985.6	1259.2	2986.4
4.39	no match	head1	243.9	1071	2086.4	3090.6
4.425	no match	head2	212.9	942.1	2066	2979.6
4.37	no match	head3	232.9	1018	2014.1	3061.2
3.72	no match	heard1	263.6	980.6	1433.9	1983.2
3.735	no match	heard2	276.8	1034	1448.3	2022.8
3.47	M-heard	heard3	263	912.5	1401	1930.4
1.134	no match	heed1	303	343.7	1770.3	2750.1
1.252	no match	heed2	303	379.4	1593.3	2959.4
1.48	no match	heed3	294.1	435.3	1667.7	2939.1
3.688	no match	hid1	244.6	902	2196	3038.8
3.502	no match	hid2	243.2	851.6	2349.6	3040.8
3.639	no match	hid3	232.3	845.3	2275.6	3006.9
2.163	no match	hood1	278.6	602.7	1202.4	2979.4
2.167	no match	hood2	278.6	603.7	1211.8	2996
3.302	no match	hud1	243.7	804.6	1327.8	2939.6
3.257	no match	hud2	243.7	793.8	1330.6	2976.3
3.269	no match	hud3	237.6	776.7	1460.1	3009.1
2.301	no match	whod1	305.9	703.8	1308.2	2955
2.119	no match	whod3	262.4	555.9	1414.3	2805.7
1/25	0.04					

Table 15 shows the results for Female Talker 1 identification using the Experiment II method. Only 4% accuracy was achieved (1 out of 25 correct), but all 24 errors involved no model match. Again, this would result in 100% accuracy with little effort. A test has showed that it is possible to achieve 100% accuracy without affecting any other results, but with only one female talker used to set the new parameters the categorical boundaries are not displayed here. The parameters would be expected to change dramatically as more female talkers are analyzed and incorporated into the model, but the demonstration that the model can be modified to account for new talkers was an important validation of how the model can be expanded to account for a wide range of individual ranges. Furthermore, the 80% accuracy rate achieved using the Experiment I method for the female talker shows the limitations of that method to account for and incorporate higher pitch productions. Additional detail could be incorporated into the Experiment I method such as utilizing F1 values in a similar fashion as is used in Experiment II to refine the categorical identification process, but this has not been achieved despite several attempts to do so. Conversely, the use of F1 in the Experiment II method became obvious when using F1/F0 to calculate the relationship between F1 and F0.

The performance exhibited using the Experiment II method compared to Experiment I shows that the method of using F1 / F0 and F1 values to categorize a vowel is more accurate and flexible than F1 – F0 / 100. Higher pitch and other variables across talkers are accounted for to a greater degree in Experiment II. Testing these three unique talkers and additional female talkers will continue to help refine the categorical boundaries and it is expected to continue to demonstrate the superior performance of the Experiment II method.

CHAPTER 5

DISCUSSION

Summary of the Experiments and Waveform Model

The finding of 93.9% correct identification in Experiment I compares well to recent results of 92% accuracy achieved by a recent spectral model of vowel perception for 45 male speakers in a perceptual study by Hillenbrand & Houde (2003). In general, the present results compare well to and surpass the perceptual results of any model attempting to perceive the American vowels across multiple talkers. Other models are comparable and do share some aspects of the parameters used in Experiment I. For example, the calculation of F1 – F0 / 100 is similar to one of the parameters used by Gopal and Syrdal (1986). They measured the distance between F1 and F0 in barks which is comparable to F1 – F0 / 100, but the similarities between the parameters of the two models ends there. Gopal and Syrdal use the barks between F2 and F1, and the barks between F3 and F2 to further distinguish a vowel from other vowels. These calculations will produce quite different results from simply using the individual F2 value as a distinguishing feature. Despite 93.9% accuracy, the method used in Experiment I was found to have serious limitations.

The method used in Experiment I was not suited for handling two males with a relatively high pitch compared to a typical male (used in this experiment), and was not suited for handling a female talker. The errors emanating from the method used in Experiment I and the inability to adjust the parameters without introducing more errors demonstrates a lack of flexibility within the model to account for this level of variability across talkers. The parameters used in Experiment I, or for that matter any model constructed using different parameters needs to account for the effects created by higher F0 values. It is possible that additional analysis using Experiment I parameters may yield better results and achieve a level of flexibility needed to account for higher pitches. However, the alternative method of calculating the ratio of F1 cycles per F0 with F1/F0 yields better results and appears to be flexible enough to account for talker variations regardless of the pitch of the talker. The F1/F0 method used in Experiment II led to an accuracy rate of 97.7%.

The 97.7% vowel identification accuracy achieved in Experiment II not only represents a 4% improvement over Experiment I, it is significantly better than any other model previously espoused in the literature. This level of performance and the ability to account for multiple talkers show a greater potential for the F1/F0 calculation and the other parameters used in Experiment II.

In Table 8, one can see that on both ends of the vowel space, the F1/F0 ratio and the F2 values are all that is required to identify the vowel. The extreme range of the ratio with a very distinctive F2 value range make additional cues unnecessary. However, in the middle of the vowel space, there is a great deal of overlap of the F1/F0 ratio resulting from the wide range in talker variability. The F2 values do occupy ranges that are distinctive, but there is still a certain amount of overlap which generates errors due to the overlapping ratio ranges created from using F1/F0. This led to the use of F1 as a cue to refine and complete the categorization of a vowel. This makes the F2 values more distinctive within the narrow categorical ranges resulting from the combined parameters of the F1/F0 ratio and F1 alone. The overlap created by using F1/F0 necessitated the need to use the additional parameter of F1 to categorize a vowel in the crowded ratio ranges, but this ratio calculation allows for a great deal more variability between talkers making the categorical boundaries wider and more flexible.

The results of Experiment II show that the method of categorizing a vowel by first establishing a general categorical range by calculating F1/F0 and then using F1 to refine the categorization is an effective categorization method. For example, the range of 2.835 to 4.3 for / U / overlaps a portion of the range for the neighboring category of vowels / æ / and / ε /. Despite the overlapping values, a vowel is clearly defined and identified by the F2 values across these overlapping categories. Furthermore, it appears that F1/F0 boundaries between vowels can be extended as long as the F2 value is clearly associated with the intended category. There is a central set of F1/F0 and F2 parameters for each vowel. The F1/F0 boundaries for each vowel can be extended or stretched to overlap with the nearest neighbor if the F2 value is made clearly enough to differentiate the vowel from the neighboring vowels with a similar F1/F0 ratio. This flexibility of the boundaries and distinguishing cues accounts for a number of talker differences including those involved with female productions.

It is interesting that the F1/F0 ratio is an important categorical cue, but F1 alone plays a significant role in a majority of categorizations. Even when F1/F0 alone is used to categorize a vowel, the unique F1 for these vowels makes this ratio distinct enough to not have the redundancy of using F1 alone. This demonstrates further the importance of the tongue positions associated with producing F1 and the lip positions associated with producing F2. Changes in pitch will change the qualitative nature of the vowel, but the tongue and lip positions will maintain the quantitative nature needed for correct identification.

Additional work is still needed, but the parameters used in Experiment II extend the level of detail initially described as the model parameters which were derived from average values reported by Peterson Barney (1952). The model is now refined and the original concept of categorizing a vowel by the F1 ratio to F0 and then distinguishing a vowel from its categorical pair with F2 continues to be the underlying foundation of this waveform model. The achievement of 97.7% accuracy rate is significant, but just as the modifications made from Experiment I to Experiment II resulted in almost a 4% increase, there are additional modifications that will be needed to achieve perfection. Because of the flexibility of the model, an eventual 100% identification rate appears to be achievable.

The parameters shown in Table 8 shows the parameters used in Experiment II and they are the final parameters for male talkers until refined by analyzing additional talkers or the correction of the errors especially between "head" and "had". The confusion errors between these two vowels accounts for 75% of the errors in Experiment II and the model produces 99% accuracy (406 out of 410) when these two vowels are eliminated from the analysis. Table 8 provides the detailed parameters the averages cannot provide, but the general framework does provide the clear patterns for categorization and distinguishing cues. From the original model based on averages, there was a method available to categorize and distinguish a vowel when specific data was available to be analyzed. The detailed measurements provided well defined parameters and additional insight into the cues that can be used to identify a vowel such as F1.

Future Work
Although additional talkers can be analyzed, at this point the most valuable data would be that obtained from a human perceptual experiment using the "head" and "had" productions used in Experi-

ment I and II as the stimuli. The most valuable result from such an experiment would be the assurance that the productions are quality productions and not ambiguous. If there are any poor productions that can be shown to be confusable by human listeners, further modifications of the Waveform Model parameters may be unnecessary since the stretching of the categorical boundary parameters may not be needed to account for a poor production. If the model is trying to account for a "head" production that is perceived as a "had" production by human listeners, this will create unnecessary overlap within the model. Even if the model has correctly identified a vowel as the intended vowel, if it is a poor production the model would benefit by not having the parameters stretched into ranges where it should not be. This could reduce some of the conditional logic currently used which would simplify the processing and improve overall performance. Finally, the focus can be on these two vowels since they currently account for 75% of the errors produced by the model.

Analyzing a significant number of female talkers beyond the one female analyzed here will extend the Waveform Model to females. Although the one female tested here was identified at 100% without adversely affecting the male identifications, the parameters used were not displayed here since the parameters will change dramatically as more females are added to the testing process. Manipulating the parameters to identify any one talker is a relatively quick process; however, the parameters of the Waveform Model are flexible enough to identify any talker including newly added talkers. The ranges that provide for that flexibility can not be established until approximately 10 talkers have been tested and analyzed. After this number of talkers there are minor adjustments, but each new talker added to the test is identified at a high rate including a rate as high as 100% the first time they are tested with the Waveform Model. This is being achieved with males, but one female can be used as an indicator of what parameters may be needed for women in general. Analyzing speech produced by children would be another step in expanding the parameters of the Waveform Model to be able to identify an English vowel regardless of age or gender the first time the values are entered into the identification test.

Beyond expanding and refining the parameters in Table 8, future work should extend the model to other portions of the vowel in a variety of coarticulatory environments. Analysis of formant values at points other than the one point in time measured at the neutral center of the vowel will need to be performed in order to identify the leading and trailing cues that can be used to identify a vowel or consonants surrounding the vowel. For example, the transition of the articulators to the positions needed to produce the /d/ at the end of the word may be reflected and identifiable in these vowels. The information of the formant patterns at the end of the vowel may be providing information about the vowel as well as the consonant /d/. If the productions were hVb (hab, hib, hob, etc.) the last third of the vowels would be expected to be unique and distinct to the /b/ as it would be for the production of /d/.

With performance at 97.7% accuracy across 20 male talkers, it is becoming evident that there is not a great deal of information that is needed beyond the formant values at the middle of the vowel in hVd productions to identify the vowel. Future work will result in improvements to the parameters, but there is also limited experimental evidence that supports another possible use of waveform analysis. Specifically, Stokes (2002) showed that waveform displays show distinguishing features that can be used to identify the talker. In two trials, a production of the word "who'd" was analyzed and used to identify that talker from a set of 10 productions of the word "who'd". Each of the 10 male productions was from a different talker, with one production being a different token of the word used as the production to be matched. The talker to be identified was correctly identified in both trials in a similar fashion as finger prints are used to identify an individual.

Talker identification has been proven to be possible by visual inspection of the complex waveform (Stokes, 2002), but just as the Waveform Model could not be supported by one individual identifying a vowel from visual displays of waveforms (Stokes, 1996, 2001) there needs to be more support for talker identification. Identifying the points of identification within waveform displays needs to be formalized and tested in a consistent and objective manner. The Waveform Model now has objective and replicable results supporting the model from the computer generated results of Experiment II. Talker identification from waveform displays will need to become formalized, in a manner similar to the process delineated in Experiment II. Because of the experimental support for talker identification from a waveform display and the success of using fingerprints as a pattern matching process to identify an individual, there is reason to be optimistic that an individual can be identified from a formal process of matching visual cues within waveform displays of the production of the same word. As with fingerprints, a known production from the person is needed to match what is suspected to have been produced by the talker. A speech segment as short as 25 to 50 milliseconds from a vowel has been shown to be all that would be required to identify a person by visually matching points within waveform displays.

Summary

Clearly, there is further potential and utility for the Waveform Model and the analysis of visual waveform displays in general. However, at present there are a number of important contributions and innovations to understanding the quality of a vowel that is currently observed in the results presented here, with 97.7% vowel identification accuracy across nine American vowels and 99% accuracy across 7 of the 9 vowels for 20 male talkers in Experiment II.

1. A new way to broadly categorize the vowel space with F1 / F0 and then refine that categorization with F1 values alone.

2. A way to distinguish between categorical pairs of vowels; differences in F2 frequencies.

3. An explanation for vowel misperceptions; categorical neighboring vowels with a similar F2 value (relatively high or low).

4. A direct link between articulatory gestures and formant frequency; tongue position with F1 and lip position with F2.

5. Vowel perception approaching human performance across talkers without the need to change parameters used for all talkers including newly introduced talkers.

6. Talker normalization is accomplished through the categorization process of F1/F0 and F1 alone.

No other model of vowel perception encompasses all of these features, and no other model has achieved 97.7% accuracy across the vowel space of nine English vowels produced by 20 male talkers. Considering that the Waveform Model can accomplish both while being relatively uncomplicated and efficient makes the features of the model more than intriguing. Furthermore, relating the relationships of articulation to specific formants from the unique categorization of the vowel space would be expected from a model that can explain human performance. The heuristically developed parameters shown in Table 8 are flexible and capable of expanding to females. No other model can accomplish these feats.

The unique features of this model are the result of a unique perspective gained from the visual relationships found in complex waveforms. The interactive relationships are not obvious from spectrogram displays that separate the formants. It has been difficult to reconstruct the relationships from the individual values, but the process described here is the reverse of the typical methods. The process in this manuscript went from a general categorization of the vowels based on the interactions perceived in waveforms and the individual values were then used to refine the categories with specific range parameters. Having the organization of the vowel space before having the specific formant values was advantageous.

This work represents a description of speech waveforms that goes beyond the limited descriptions found previously in the literature. During the description of waveforms, a new model of vowel perception and vowel production has been detailed. The 97.7% accuracy rate achieved in an objective and reproducible experiment currently stands alone compared to other vowel perception models in the literature.

REFERENCES

Avaaz Innovations, Inc. (1998). TFR, the Time Frequency Representation software, version 3.0. Avaaz Innovations Inc,, 1225 Wonderland Road North, London, Ontario, N6G 2B0, Canada (http://www.avaaz.com).

Chiba, T. and Kajiyama, J. (1941). *The vowel: its nature and structure.* Tokyo: Tokyo-Kaisekan Publishing Co.

Cole, R.A., Rudnicky, A.I., & Zue, V.W. (1979). Performance of an expert spectrogram reader. In *Speech Communication Papers Presented at the 97th Meeting of the Acoustical Society of America,* edited by J.J. Wolf and D.H. Klatt (Acoustical Society of America, New York, NY).

Cole, R., and Zue, V. (1980). *Speech as Eyes See it* (pp. 475-494). In Attention and Performance VIII, Hillsdale, NJ: Lawrence Erlbaum Assoc.

Hillenbrand, J. and Houde, R. (2003). A narrow band pattern-matching model of vowel perception, *Journal of the Acoustical Society of America, 113,* 1044–1055.

Hubbard, B. B. (1998). *The world according to wavelets: The story of a mathematical technique in the making.* Natick, MA: AK Peters, Ltd.

Jamieson, D.G., Ramji, K., Kheirallah, I., & Nearey, T.M. (1992). CSRE: A speech research environment. ICSLP-1992, 1127-1130.

Klatt, D.H. (1988). Review of selected models of speech perception. In W.D. Marslen-Wilson (Ed.), *Lexical representation and process* (pp. 201-262). Cambridge, MA: MIT Press.

Ladefoged, P. (1982). *A course in phonetics,* New York, NY: Harcourt Brace Jovanovich.

Mullennix, J.W. (1994). Midwestern Talker Database.

Peterson, G.E., & Barney, H.L. (1952). Control methods used in the study of vowels, *Journal of the Acoustical Society of America, 24,* 175–84.

Scott, B.L. (1980). Speech as patterns in time. In R.A. Cole (Ed.), *Perception and production of fluent speech* (pp. 51-70). Hillsdale, NJ: Ealbaum.

Stokes, M.A. (1996). Identification of vowels based on visual cues within raw complex waveforms. Paper presented at the 131st meeting of the Acoustical Society of America.

Stokes, M.A. (2001). Male and female vowels identified by visual inspection of raw complex waveforms. Paper presented at the 141st meeting of the Acoustical Society of America.

Stokes, M.A. (2002). Talker identification from analysis of raw complex waveforms. Paper presented at the 143rd Meeting of the Acoustical Society of America, June, Pittsburgh, PA.

Summers, W.V., Pisoni, D.B., Bernacki, R.H., Pedlow, R.I., & Stokes, M.A. (1988). Effects of noise on speech production: Acoustic and perceptual analysis. Journal of the Acoustical Society of America, 84, 917-928.

Summers, W.V., Pisoni, D.B., and Stokes M.A. (1989), Effects of cognitive workload on speech production. Paper presented at the 117th meeting: Acoustical Society of America, May, Syracuse, NY.

The measurements taken for each production by each talker used in Experiment I and II is displayed in this appendix. The tables display the F0, F1, F2, and F3 measurements and the time at which the measurements were taken. The number associated with the vowel is the token for that vowel for that talker. The ratio is calculated from F1/F0 and the entire table for each talker is ordered by these calculations.

Male Talker 1

Vowel	Ratio	F0 value	F1 value	F2 value	F3 value	Time
heed3	2.091027	153.8	321.6	2351	2915.9	522
heed1	2.158416	151.5	327	2553	3000	581
heed2	2.287095	144.9	331.4	2451.4	2952.6	480
whod2	2.453193	161.3	395.7	1125.5	2383.6	533
whod1	2.866711	149.3	428	1078	2427.7	400
whod3	2.944935	147.1	433.2	1078.8	2303.8	585
hid2	3.272727	140.8	460.8	1993.5	2670.8	510
hood3	3.615908	147.1	531.9	1218.8	2496.3	544
hood2	3.730849	144.9	540.6	1171.4	2540.3	555
hid1	3.70219	137	507.2	1958.8	2671.3	355
heard2	3.891223	133.3	518.7	1401.4	1634	1007
heard3	3.894161	137	533.5	1369.5	1671.4	453
hid3	3.879349	135.1	524.1	1929	2583.3	450
hood1	4.169767	129	537.9	1223.7	2546.5	255
heard1	4.146266	129.9	538.6	1423.4	1734.9	734
hud3	4.994749	133.3	665.8	1272.2	2613.9	580
hud2	5.007502	133.3	667.5	1338.5	2634.7	375
head2	5.036182	129.9	654.2	1804.1	2565.4	640
head1	5.047112	131.6	664.2	1733.3	2588.5	373
hud1	5.165512	129.9	671	1341.7	2622.6	463
head3	5.155608	126.6	652.7	1762.4	2524.1	490
had3	5.1656	125	645.7	1873.9	2500.3	552
had1	5.2952	125	661.9	1873.9	2464.9	650
had2	5.617077	113.6	638.1	1878.5	2505.8	686
hawed3	5.893927	123.5	727.9	1026.9	2804.8	716
hawed2	6.224278	135.1	840.9	1078.6	2766.4	970
hawed1	6.369842	133.3	849.1	1098.1	2714	454

Male Talker 2

Vowel	Ratio	F0 value	F1 value	F2 value	F3 value	Time
whod2	2.055302	175.4	360.5	1236.3	2159.2	547
heed3	2.136541	153.8	328.6	2250.1	2862.4	791
heed1	2.145558	158.7	340.5	2338.5	2881.4	416
heed2	2.330083	133.3	310.6	2263.9	3008.8	610
whod1	2.580292	137	353.5	1147.9	2136.4	638
whod3	3.082067	131.6	405.6	1183.4	2114.7	733
hid2	3.15597	144.9	457.3	1961.7	2638.7	763
heard3	3.288011	149.3	490.9	1296.2	1672.7	825
hood2	3.32155	147.1	488.6	1145.3	2297.2	754
hood1	3.354356	153.8	515.9	1132.9	2321.7	572
hid3	3.465046	131.6	456	1902.2	2493.9	888
heard2	3.676292	131.6	483.8	1346.4	1686.6	830
heard1	3.610795	140.8	508.4	1327.6	1696.6	835
hood3	3.771533	137	516.7	1130.2	2292.8	982
hid1	4.1	122	500.2	1904.5	2575	567
head2	4.316062	135.1	583.1	1837.4	2436.8	750
head1	4.558511	131.6	599.9	1838.2	2418.2	700
hud3	4.863805	135.1	657.1	1252	2367.3	701
hud2	4.938564	135.1	667.2	1276.1	2419.9	1109
had2	5.0336	125	629.2	1937.5	2377.3	450
hawed2	5.036474	131.6	662.8	1082.9	2321.5	510
had3	5.099526	126.6	645.6	1934.5	2386.3	567
head3	5.1768	125	647.1	1810.2	2379.4	783
hud1	5.242496	126.6	663.7	1246.5	2445.1	573
hawed3	5.801619	123.5	716.5	1113.6	2319.3	800
hawed1	5.942623	122	725	1117.5	2326.8	810

Male Talker 3

Vowel	Ratio	F0 value	F1 value	F2 value	F3 value	Time
heed3	2.026316	178.6	361.9	2322.8	2797.5	604
heed2	2.062714	175.4	361.8	2359.5	3181.2	634
whod2	2.020668	188.7	381.3	964.4	2284.7	560
heed1	2.0028	178.6	357.7	2352	3147	690
whod3	2.172166	166.7	362.1	1033	2264.3	700
hid2	2.984598	181.8	542.6	1845.5	2786.1	600
hood2	3.092382	166.7	515.5	1049.1	2496.5	649
hid1	3.091491	156.3	483.2	1858.4	2529.6	620
hid3	3.168317	151.5	480	1873.3	2577.6	850
heard1	3.230409	149.3	482.3	1261.7	1632.5	1023
hood3	3.370395	149.3	503.2	1107.2	2527.2	630
heard2	3.435078	147.1	505.3	1254.4	1616.4	595
heard3	3.841613	138.9	533.6	1303	1725.5	455
hud3	4.147354	149.3	619.2	1195.2	2660.5	570
hud1	4.846791	144.9	702.3	1125	2566.1	742
hud2	4.80438	137	658.2	1155.3	2598.4	566
head1	4.911222	140.8	691.5	1703.3	2436.7	590
hawed3	4.992598	135.1	674.5	986	2758.6	610
head3	5.074759	135.1	685.6	1679.3	2531.6	469
head2	5.053276	138.9	701.9	1661.6	2408.7	1130
hawed2	5.024961	128.2	644.2	1028.2	2505.1	680
had3	5.119345	128.2	656.3	1806	2438.8	770
had2	5.111769	135.1	690.6	1898.8	2400	603

Male Talker 4

Vowel	Ratio	F0 value	F1 value	F2 value	F3 value	Time
heed1	2.255349	144.9	326.8	2350.1	3013.1	344
heed2	2.352694	142.9	336.2	2310.9	2953.3	1252
whod1	2.328614	169.5	394.7	984.7	2449.7	986
whod3	2.455787	153.8	377.7	948.5	2455.6	1171
whod2	2.594059	151.5	393	931.4	2465.4	1599
heed3	2.690531	129.9	349.5	2307.8	3017.3	798
hid3	3.236506	140.8	455.7	1991.4	2807.3	959
hid2	3.775212	129.9	490.4	1945.1	2739.1	1100
hood3	3.866477	140.8	544.4	1209.8	2622.1	777
hood1	3.927737	137	538.1	1258.2	2553.7	602
hood2	4.033008	133.3	537.6	1250.5	2568.3	820
heard2	4.108068	135.1	555	1297.5	1728.9	1170
hid1	4.1816	125	522.7	1917.3	2734.7	662
heard1	4.251639	122	518.7	1367.2	1808.5	823
heard3	4.297976	123.5	530.8	1341.1	1804.9	965
hud3	4.787899	147.1	704.3	1269.7	2758	1779
hud2	4.907727	133.3	654.2	1230.9	2761.7	1082
head2	5.027737	137	688.8	1699.6	2761.3	1123
head1	5.073153	140.8	714.3	1658.2	2617.8	1300
had3	5.1712	125	646.4	1886.8	2663.9	860
head3	5.409647	138.9	751.4	1700.9	2693.7	1170
hud1	5.504876	133.3	733.8	1298.1	2792.8	1343
had2	5.721169	126.6	724.3	1839.1	2631	880
hawed3	5.87358	140.8	827	1100	2799.2	1160
hawed2	5.87067	129.9	762.6	1162.3	2821.2	723
had1	5.806557	122	708.4	1842.5	2621.7	976
hawed1	6.395529	116.3	743.8	1107.3	2780.9	1860

Male Talker 5

Vowel	Ratio	F0 value	F1 value	F2 value	F3 value	Time
heed1	1.982004	166.7	330.4	2158.5	3172.4	670
heed3	2.031268	169.5	344.3	2108.1	2951.2	458
whod3	2.06271	178.6	368.4	1071.3	2214.2	555
heed2	2.066336	161.3	333.3	2305.7	3268.2	763
whod2	2.031915	178.6	362.9	1017.3	2274.1	501
whod1	2.030207	188.7	383.1	1089.5	2298.4	629
hid3	2.87645	172.4	495.9	1885.8	2462.9	965
hid2	2.997399	153.8	461	1844	2579.6	572
heard3	3.051184	156.3	476.9	1440.8	1680.8	810
hood2	3.070056	161.3	495.2	1172.9	2498.3	821
hood1	3.042591	166.7	507.2	1165.7	2515.4	661
heard2	3.202947	149.3	478.2	1379.5	1718.7	467
hid1	3.277178	138.9	455.2	1837.9	2566.1	843
heard1	3.307299	137	453.1	1364.7	1680.2	916
hood3	3.586738	149.3	535.5	1226.2	2369.5	849
hud2	3.986137	158.7	632.6	1131.6	2561.7	843
head1	4.197589	149.3	626.7	1659.5	2566.1	642
head3	4.282294	158.7	679.6	1644.1	2494.6	527
hud1	4.354861	147.1	640.6	1044.1	2554.8	636
head2	4.599034	144.9	666.4	1613.4	2516	455
hawed3	4.549415	153.8	699.7	1058.5	2607.5	570
had3	4.556934	137	624.3	1856.6	2493.9	539
hud3	4.632979	131.6	609.7	1149.2	2534.4	390
hawed1	4.660066	151.5	706	1068.9	2613.9	474
hawed2	4.751575	142.9	679	1007.7	2647	628
had2	4.715328	137	646	1779.8	2483.6	545
had1	4.84452	117.7	570.2	1834.1	2512.7	755

Male Talker 6

Vowel	Ratio	F0 value	F1 value	F2 value	F3 value	Time
heed2	2.064369	153.8	317.5	2422	2967.6	310
heed1	2.019142	151.5	305.9	2422.3	2872.7	390
heed3	2.161491	144.9	313.2	2385	2868.7	404
whod2	2.642909	138.9	367.1	1350.1	2486.7	230
whod3	2.617822	151.5	396.6	1301.2	2401.2	545
heard1	2.752177	149.3	410.9	1457.1	1760.1	1980
whod1	2.734762	149.3	408.3	1337.8	2406.9	220
hood1	3.057583	175.4	536.3	1438.2	2399.5	555
hid3	3.050715	153.8	469.2	1958	2520	1163
hid1	3.095238	144.9	448.5	2000.8	2570.3	283
heard2	3.290483	140.8	463.3	1405.8	1777.2	290
heard3	3.39635	137	465.3	1427.7	1761.2	390
hid2	3.519078	138.9	488.8	1972	2570.2	245
hood2	3.658771	135.1	494.3	1501.9	2438.3	304
hood3	3.979745	133.3	530.5	1389.1	2394.1	522
head1	4.156731	149.3	620.6	1813.8	2601.9	151
hud3	4.637509	142.9	662.7	1315.5	2221.6	949
hud2	4.771943	133.3	636.1	1364.3	2225.1	591
had3	4.753188	133.3	633.6	1933.4	2502.9	220
had2	4.798668	135.1	648.3	1968.7	2538.8	440
hud1	4.890995	126.6	619.2	1376	2369.3	445
head3	4.835549	142.9	691	1834.9	2560.8	250
head2	4.857883	135.1	656.3	1775.6	2556.5	250
had1	4.973479	128.2	637.6	1923.7	2463.7	415
hawed2	5.50073	137	753.6	1246.9	2595	256
hawed3	5.941489	131.6	781.9	1231.9	2667.1	460
hawed1	6.088522	133.3	811.6	1266.7	2636.8	1540

Male Talker 7

Vowel	Ratio	F0 value	F1 value	F2 value	F3 value	Time
whod2	1.4308	250	357.7	730.8	1804.7	770
whod1	1.6532	250	413.3	721.1	1822.8	1875
heed3	1.824747	217.4	396.7	2218.4	2872.1	1003
heard1	1.806188	294.1	531.2	1334.3	1761.8	577
heed2	1.899069	204.1	387.6	2281.7	3024.7	617
whod3	1.89739	222.2	421.6	634.9	2090.3	635
heed1	1.9245	200	384.9	2319.6	2920.4	735
hid2	2.239098	204.1	457	2000.2	2429.2	598
hid3	2.3545	200	470.9	1973.3	2465.8	939
hid1	2.3845	200	476.9	1996.2	2479	1049
hood3	2.360902	212.8	502.4	1389.3	2265.4	729
heard2	2.591455	208.3	539.8	1270.9	1692.8	831
hood1	2.606783	188.7	491.9	1039.5	2310.5	688
hood2	2.767819	185.2	512.6	1198.9	2235.4	1126
heard3	2.836713	192.3	545.5	1366.6	1726.9	509
head3	2.994701	188.7	565.1	1883.3	2421.7	805
head2	3.060475	185.2	566.8	1878.8	2423.2	2249
head1	3.142691	172.4	541.8	1935.8	2568.1	905
had2	3.397816	192.3	653.4	1940.3	2465.7	771
hud2	3.650715	181.8	663.7	1200.2	2359.7	2189
hawed2	3.690065	185.2	683.4	887.3	2403.6	735
hud3	3.645215	181.8	662.7	1178.7	2264.7	898
had1	3.892497	178.6	695.2	1930.7	2409.8	850
hawed1	3.81299	178.6	681	888	2541.3	1634
hud1	3.932153	169.5	666.5	1231.2	2365.9	960
hawed3	3.932155	175.4	689.7	1017.1	2441.7	777
had3	3.982599	172.4	686.6	1907.9	2445.7	640

Male Talker 8

Vowel	Ratio	F0 value	F1 value	F2 value	F3 value	Time
heed3	2.040947	156.3	319	2441.5	3215.8	579
heed2	2.067301	147.1	304.1	2439.9	3185.2	664
heed1	2.018466	140.8	284.2	2347.5	3256.8	1157
whod3	2.198504	147.1	323.4	959.2	2470.3	1146
whod1	2.25943	129.9	293.5	951.5	2470.4	2476
whod2	2.333827	135.1	315.3	964.5	2603.2	599
had2	2.5	250	625	2015.8	2532.8	771
hid3	2.658385	144.9	385.2	2210.7	2723.9	635
hood3	2.988958	144.9	433.1	1465.3	2510.6	642
hid2	2.985746	133.3	398	2292.6	2844.3	1466
hid1	2.942265	135.1	397.5	2290.6	2759.1	596
hood1	3.154255	131.6	415.1	1476.1	2585.8	1226
hood2	3.239021	138.9	449.9	1477.5	2530.4	1115
heard1	3.7528	125	469.1	1446.2	1592.7	1258
heard3	3.771307	140.8	531	1390.8	1859.4	720
heard2	3.821455	133.3	509.4	1449.5	1807	741
head3	3.931108	140.8	553.5	2074.9	2693.7	636
head1	3.979275	135.1	537.6	2143.2	2611.9	1120
hud3	4.312455	138.9	599	1444.6	2517.5	866
hud2	4.636644	129.9	602.3	1439.2	2572.8	846
hawed2	4.764619	135.1	643.7	1118.6	2555.4	1072
had3	4.723722	140.8	665.1	1966.8	2447.6	539
hawed3	4.80681	135.1	649.4	1076.1	2565.5	770
hud1	4.9952	125	624.4	1411.1	2652.4	705
had1	5.015544	135.1	677.6	1954.2	3446.6	816
hawed1	5.223404	131.6	687.4	1080.6	2678.5	936

Male Talker 9

Vowel	Ratio	F0 value	F1 value	F2 value	F3 value	Time
heed2	1.845895	208.3	384.5	2562.4	3578.1	881
heed1	1.986659	172.4	342.5	2575.5	3594.8	1178
whod2	2.030238	185.2	376	1134	2264.9	1183
heed3	2.10397	158.7	333.9	2449.8	3597.9	685
whod1	2.289201	163.9	375.2	1140.2	2189.8	1072
whod3	2.301156	147.1	338.5	1071.8	2369.1	791
heard3	2.401244	192.9	463.2	1210.9	1533.2	996
heard2	3.06567	153.8	471.5	1328.5	1701.9	617
hood1	3.067724	163.9	502.8	1321.9	2209.6	1180
hid1	3.063453	163.9	502.1	1919.7	2396.4	1491
hood3	3.041392	166.7	507	1321.7	2089.8	935
hid2	3.115735	153.8	479.2	1897.1	2404.7	624
heard1	3.228433	144.9	467.8	1301.3	1637.6	1214
hood2	3.273275	149.3	488.7	1306.4	2178.3	783
hid3	3.49815	135.1	472.6	1842	2381.3	1547
head2	3.957902	144.9	573.5	1696.8	2451.4	1373
hud2	4.044991	166.7	674.3	1227.1	2460.7	1234
head1	4.080624	153.8	627.6	1693.4	2307.2	978
hud1	4.280234	153.8	658.3	1294.4	2360.4	1018
had3	4.981377	123.5	615.2	1781.2	2287.8	568
head3	4.92123	133.3	656	1744.6	2328.3	676
hawed3	5.07624	135.1	685.8	1081.9	2486.4	771
hud3	5.1406	126.6	650.8	1244.3	2222.7	555
had1	5.131556	116.3	596.8	1844.2	2181.9	611
hawed2	5.142097	131.6	676.7	1017.7	2453.9	747
hawed1	5.132619	149.3	766.3	1161.1	2506	439
had2	5.169267	128.2	662.7	1928.2	2299.4	1999

Male Talker 10

Vowel	Ratio	F0 value	F1 value	F2 value	F3 value	Time
heed3	1.952883	161.3	315	2276.3	2816.4	804
heed2	2.029147	188.7	382.9	2297.6	2799.9	1138
whod2	2.043682	192.3	393	1184.1	2301.5	1481
heed1	2.017488	188.7	380.7	2373.2	2866.8	825
whod1	2.061555	185.2	381.8	1123.6	2249.7	2162
whod3	2.243039	172.4	386.7	1200.2	2224.6	749
hid1	2.801044	172.4	482.9	1879.3	2552.9	1154
hid2	2.865627	166.7	477.7	1834.8	2507.7	736
heard3	2.950728	178.6	527	1441.9	1821.8	939
hood1	2.923037	192.3	562.1	1198.3	2491.8	1086
hood2	2.968073	175.4	520.6	1241.5	2466.3	1333
hid3	2.958412	158.7	469.5	1830.5	2582.6	1044
heard1	3.065545	172.4	528.5	1427.2	1768	3413
heard2	3.066336	161.3	494.6	1471.1	1786.2	773
head2	3.789417	185.2	701.8	1647	2557.6	1755
head3	3.832953	175.4	672.3	1630.6	2557.1	1082
hud1	3.909263	158.7	620.4	1216.8	2582.9	1582
hud2	4.058086	151.5	614.8	1215	2627.2	1200
hood3	4.012753	133.3	534.9	1200.3	2518.9	944
head1	4.018596	166.7	669.9	1683.7	2533.9	1198
hawed2	4.497795	158.7	713.8	1122.3	2565.5	1642
hud3	4.515328	137	618.6	1326.8	2577.6	2060
had1	4.636302	147.1	682	1890.8	2581.3	1283
hawed1	4.637624	151.5	702.6	980.6	2666.1	811
had3	4.759972	142.9	680.2	1844.4	2546.2	800
had2	4.899858	140.8	689.9	1817.8	2553.5	965
hawed3	4.910945	147.1	722.4	1155.2	2639.5	1032

Male Talker 12

Vowel	Ratio	F0 value	F1 value	F2 value	F3 value	Time
whod3	1.852107	232.6	430.8	935.2	2324.2	1933
heed2	1.983759	172.4	342	2193.5	2812.5	436
heed3	2.035398	169.5	345	2240.3	2853	1102
whod1	2.029675	178.6	362.5	887.5	2207.2	1701
whod2	2.012318	178.6	359.4	1078.5	2173.4	1820
heed1	2.037828	163.9	334	2166.5	2970.8	780
hid3	2.582891	169.5	437.8	1953.8	2608.1	1659
hid2	2.770246	166.7	461.8	1945.6	2612.8	1134
heard3	2.85123	166.7	475.3	1358.1	1574.6	611
hid1	2.868822	163.9	470.2	1857.1	2506.2	1160
heard1	2.919405	161.3	470.9	1325.9	1545.5	1399
hood1	2.943868	163.9	482.5	1149.4	2393.5	213
had3	3.137471	172.4	540.9	2017.4	2522.4	1618
hood3	3.137954	151.5	475.4	1137.9	2457.8	1245
hood2	3.121452	151.5	472.9	1055.9	2410.6	676
heard2	3.546353	131.6	466.7	1415.6	1576.2	1088
hud1	3.898719	163.9	639	1146.7	2464.2	2182
had2	3.846858	163.9	630.5	1967.7	2449.8	1395
head3	3.933949	140.8	553.9	1619.2	2477.3	488
head2	3.968729	147.1	583.8	1715.4	2579.7	1160
head1	3.910945	147.1	575.3	1725	2513.2	1340
hud3	4.008957	156.3	626.6	1109.6	2541.7	623
hud2	4.035499	149.3	602.5	1114.1	2530.1	1723
had1	4.027872	147.1	592.5	1898	2438.8	917
hawed3	4.115512	181.8	748.2	1083.8	2640.8	2210
hawed2	4.30297	151.5	651.9	909.3	2654.7	1866
hawed1	5.205626	149.3	777.2	1070.7	2603.1	1250

Male Talker 13

Vowel	Ratio	F0 value	F1 value	F2 value	F3 value	Time
heed2	1.964239	153.8	302.1	2531.4	3242.1	514
heed3	2.022103	149.3	301.9	2443.5	3344.7	452
heed1	2.009901	151.5	304.5	2468.4	3332.6	373
whod1	2.092628	158.7	332.1	1126	2636.2	454
whod2	2.110129	147.1	310.4	1122.3	2570.8	518
whod3	2.587473	138.9	359.4	1010.6	2526.7	551
hid2	3.072993	137	421	2058.6	2705	522
hid3	3.045985	137	417.3	2118.3	2796	378
heard1	3.157036	147.1	464.4	1606.8	1941.5	783
heard3	3.465805	131.6	456.1	1497.3	1847.7	498
hood2	3.797449	133.3	506.2	1347.1	2659.5	577
hid1	3.9088	125	488.6	2060.1	2756.9	411
hood3	4.009623	135.1	541.7	1392.6	2494.9	514
heard2	4.092946	120.5	493.2	1647.7	2235.4	599
hood1	4.00624	128.2	513.6	1325.3	2576.7	600
hud2	4.694301	135.1	634.2	1398	2515.9	773
hud1	4.791937	138.9	665.6	1420.7	2543.9	831
hud3	4.836193	128.2	620	1387	2465	500
had1	4.986861	137	683.2	1967.6	2577.8	829
head2	5.101275	133.3	680	1784.4	2628.3	1338
had2	5.323065	126.6	673.9	2010.3	2657.5	595
hawed1	5.428467	137	743.7	1167.5	2513.6	630
hawed2	5.721169	126.6	724.3	1154.4	2586.1	309
head1	5.837723	117.7	687.1	1794.2	2678.8	875
head3	5.885477	120.5	709.2	1883.5	2703.9	305
hawed3	5.9696	125	746.2	1132.1	2703.5	578
had3	5.984523	116.3	696	2007.9	2615.5	419

Male Talker 15

Vowel	Ratio	F0 value	F1 value	F2 value	F3 value	Time
heed3	1.942391	208.3	404.6	2495.9	3013.5	880
heed2	1.933957	192.3	371.9	2495.8	2906.3	1139
whod3	1.976541	217.4	429.7	881.5	2391.7	742
whod1	1.908004	217.4	414.8	867.4	2362.8	1423
heed1	2.028194	166.7	338.1	2603	3054.1	2573
whod2	2.011759	204.1	410.6	822	2126.6	955
heard2	2.697868	192.3	518.8	1251.8	1595.5	1044
hood2	2.7705	200	554.1	1212.3	2405.6	1423
hid1	2.723872	181.8	495.2	1993.4	2683.1	1564
hid3	2.912594	212.8	619.8	1919.7	2478	924
hid2	2.984102	188.7	563.1	1906.3	2587.7	2075
had2	3.086393	185.2	571.6	2128.7	2664.8	964
heard1	3.170321	196.1	621.7	1218.3	1572	1866
heard3	3.276825	204.1	668.8	1299.1	1710.5	870
hood3	3.226729	192.3	620.5	1218.8	2440	1275
hood1	3.30108	222.2	733.5	1248.6	2269.4	841
hud3	3.9345	200	786.9	1284.7	2401.8	933
hud1	3.954647	178.6	706.3	1272.3	2380.4	948
hud2	3.984881	185.2	738	1312.5	2442.3	1166
head3	4.09681	181.8	744.8	1966.4	2755.4	1600
had3	4.030787	175.4	707	2072.8	2769.7	1797
had1	4.055451	158.7	643.6	2094.9	2665.4	1380
head1	4.691489	131.6	617.4	1827.4	2551.4	1280
hawed2	4.987204	156.3	779.5	1175.8	2447.4	1295
hawed3	5.119002	156.3	800.1	1228.8	2432.2	959

Male Talker 16

Vowel	Ratio	F0 value	F1 value	F2 value	F3 value	Time
heed3	1.993521	185.2	369.2	2093.3	2652.4	1177
whod3	1.993281	178.6	356	754.8	2162.1	1049
heed2	2.051251	163.9	336.2	2174.7	2791.3	1417
whod2	2.08691	188.7	393.8	967.5	2160.9	1277
whod1	2.077286	169.5	352.1	895.7	2158.9	1987
heed1	2.126984	144.9	308.2	2182.1	2732.1	1880
heard2	2.856103	178.6	510.1	1336.5	1667.1	1204
hood3	2.961496	181.8	538.4	1150.5	2236.6	1576
hid3	2.965974	158.7	470.7	1730.9	2469.6	1134
hid2	2.954123	161.3	476.5	1809.2	2444.8	1399
hid1	2.950442	169.5	500.1	1667.3	2383.2	1306
heard3	3.022575	163.9	495.4	1314.8	1657.7	1779
hood2	3.091519	163.9	506.7	1174.2	2349.3	1367
hud2	3.092959	181.8	562.3	1292.5	2433.4	1321
hood1	3.213545	163.9	526.7	1211.9	2343.8	2694
head3	3.407773	172.4	587.5	1594.2	2389.2	1422
hawed2	3.712657	175.4	651.2	1022.7	2586.4	1136
hud3	3.95241	163.9	647.8	1267.4	2518.1	1438
hud1	3.962802	161.3	639.2	1247	2516.7	1650
head1	3.927536	158.7	623.3	1613	2418	1509
had2	4.371771	158.7	693.8	1649.9	2377.3	1108
head2	4.560532	142.9	651.7	1520.6	2384.9	1505
hawed3	4.76069	133.3	634.6	1001.2	2567.4	1813
had3	5.17244	129.9	671.9	1679.9	2367.9	1233
had1	5.122465	128.2	656.7	1687.9	2393.7	1008
hawed1	5.21485	126.6	660.2	982.4	2634.7	2012

Male Talker 17

Vowel	Ratio	F0 value	F1 value	F2 value	F3 value	Time
heed3	1.985603	166.7	331	2215.8	3226.6	855
heed1	1.951023	161.3	314.7	2114.1	2997.4	821
whod3	1.946004	185.2	360.4	903.5	2143.5	953
heed2	2.027958	153.8	311.9	2175.9	2809.5	704
whod2	2.070775	163.9	339.4	1002.3	2166.3	761
whod1	2.030088	169.5	344.1	1024.4	2108.3	801
heard2	2.983095	153.8	458.8	1414.9	1637.4	738
hid2	2.99937	158.7	476	1849.1	2484.7	842
hid1	2.987274	149.3	446	1874.6	2484.9	702
hood3	3.032858	161.3	489.2	1165	2453.7	751
hood2	3.005041	158.7	476.9	1245.9	2373.7	877
heard1	3.141254	151.5	475.9	1413.7	1601.2	762
heard3	3.136069	138.9	435.6	1392.7	1608.9	567
hid3	3.255064	133.3	433.9	1851.5	2510.9	480
hood1	3.387097	133.3	451.5	1186.7	2250.8	1635
hud1	4.051365	153.8	623.1	1134.6	2594	862
head2	4.031271	147.1	593	1777	2497.3	878
head1	4.091749	151.5	619.9	1789.2	2531.1	981
had1	4.870739	140.8	685.8	1822	2438.3	898
hud3	4.914894	131.6	646.8	1185.3	2559.8	1006
hawed3	4.910437	135.1	663.4	1003.6	2619.2	686
had3	5.098632	138.9	708.2	1756.1	2444.1	897
head3	5.130265	128.2	657.7	1720.2	2435	767
had2	5.116225	128.2	655.9	1842.8	2471.8	734
hud2	5.2416	125	655.2	1102.7	2475.3	1578
hawed2	5.56351	129.9	722.7	1022.2	2563.3	800
hawed1	5.914189	117.7	696.1	1040.3	2602.3	825

Male Talker 18

Vowel	Ratio	F0 value	F1 value	F2 value	F3 value	Time
heed2	2.0062	161.3	323.6	2315.6	3167.9	592
heed1	2.09277	156.3	327.1	2308.2	3152.5	760
whod1	2.018205	153.8	310.4	738.2	2344.4	647
whod2	2.137307	149.3	319.1	960.1	2378.6	555
heed3	2.115328	137	289.8	2251.4	2969.2	599
whod3	2.203744	138.9	306.1	883.6	2386.7	551
hid1	3.183575	144.9	461.3	1887.9	2619.7	696
hid2	3.487054	142.9	498.3	1886.6	2668.6	462
hid3	3.670668	133.3	489.3	1866	2617.3	700
heard1	3.725389	135.1	503.3	1257.8	1538.1	1666
heard3	3.99928	138.9	555.5	1300.1	1617.9	816
hood1	3.960403	138.9	550.1	1078.1	2638.3	810
hood3	4.028798	138.9	559.6	1170.1	2616.7	692
hood2	4.141377	135.1	559.5	1122.2	2647.6	584
heard2	4.167213	122	508.4	1377.7	1657.3	638
hud3	4.373723	137	599.2	1182	2755.4	701
hud2	4.711325	135.1	636.5	1148.6	2736.3	508
hud1	4.951368	131.6	651.6	1095.6	2820.5	839
head1	5.115529	133.3	681.9	1691	2654.9	511
had1	5.359422	131.6	705.3	1976.7	2714.5	820
head2	5.387991	129.9	699.9	1612.3	2645.9	581
had3	5.597571	123.5	691.3	1943.9	2557.1	756
hawed1	5.840164	122	712.5	1108.6	2875.1	557
head3	5.931181	117.7	698.1	1627.8	2590.6	563
hawed3	6.068819	117.7	714.3	1046.1	2823.2	654
hawed2	6.170901	129.9	801.6	1047.2	2898	394
had2	6.212382	116.3	722.5	1881.2	2687.6	276

Male Talker 19

Vowel	Ratio	F0 value	F1 value	F2 value	F3 value	Time
heed3	1.975688	156.3	308.8	2274.9	3142.6	476
heed2	1.952414	142.9	279	2342.4	3218	462
whod2	2.00462	151.5	303.7	928.2	2316.5	402
heed1	2.013296	142.9	287.7	2264.7	3305.5	539
whod1	2.053966	153.8	315.9	952.8	2219.7	328
whod3	2.251095	137	308.4	1098.5	2283.8	342
hid2	2.933379	147.1	431.5	2038.8	2615.5	377
hid1	2.953093	147.1	434.4	1989.6	2554.1	487
hood3	3.059035	138.9	424.9	1254.2	2323.4	513
hid3	3.043197	138.9	422.7	1978.5	2619.4	475
hood1	3.559282	128.2	456.3	1142.7	2181	511
heard3	3.757009	117.7	442.2	1258	1503.7	1158
hood2	3.861411	120.5	465.3	1208.3	2264.9	604
heard1	3.891597	119	463.1	1166.3	1417.6	385
heard2	3.91906	114.9	450.3	1163	1425.6	982
head3	4.068267	133.3	542.3	1929.6	2527.6	421
head1	4.101106	126.6	519.2	1876.7	2444.2	923
head2	4.7744	125	596.8	1837.3	2454.9	326
hawed1	4.931162	135.1	666.2	1044.1	2092.1	414
had1	5.152931	117.7	606.5	2009.4	3681.4	337
hud2	5.321162	120.5	641.2	1287.3	2300.2	363
hud1	5.497479	119	654.2	1208.8	2265.3	139
had3	5.464186	107.5	587.4	1913	2457.3	475
had2	5.454462	108.7	592.9	1982	2473.3	383
hawed3	5.6248	125	703.1	1059.7	2225.7	287
hud3	5.736655	112.4	644.8	1243.9	2298.9	349

Male Talker 20

Vowel	Ratio	F0 value	F1 value	F2 value	F3 value	Time
whod2	1.775	200	355	990.3	2123.7	390
whod1	1.832783	181.8	333.2	1072.2	2250.4	951
heed3	2.135766	137	292.6	2302.6	2986.8	1127
heed2	2.136259	129.9	277.5	2405.1	3166.4	402
heed1	2.111769	135.1	285.3	2437.9	3098.3	1775
whod3	2.308029	137	316.2	969.6	2206.4	487
hid3	2.989921	138.9	415.3	2078.6	2715.6	1070
heard1	3.463616	133.3	461.7	1192.3	1494.4	781
hood1	3.539271	123.5	437.1	1108.9	2307.7	736
heard3	3.79895	133.3	506.4	1303.6	1616.2	457
hood3	3.797192	128.2	486.8	1120.3	2348.3	520
hid2	3.794262	122	462.9	1986.1	2706.9	1759
hid1	3.959336	120.5	477.1	1999.1	2756.8	860
hood2	4.04418	117.7	476	1160.8	2234.2	1000
heard2	4.30423	111.1	478.2	1332.9	1588.1	1816
hud1	4.791378	129.9	622.4	1227.5	2536.2	692
had1	4.942263	129.9	642	1948.6	2508.5	1059
hud2	5.028081	128.2	644.6	1282.7	2420.4	1771
hud3	5.057662	126.6	640.3	1242.5	2254	928
head2	5.27479	119	627.7	1804.9	2682.7	870
head1	5.244813	120.5	632	1804.9	2818.5	790
had2	5.676698	116.3	660.2	1933.8	2573.5	725
had3	5.708185	112.4	641.6	1893.5	2588.1	1057
hawed3	5.848667	116.3	680.2	992.4	2470.8	1212
hawed2	6.100534	112.4	685.7	960.5	2529.9	715
hawed1	6.20342	111.1	689.2	1053.8	2334.5	1130

Male Talker 22

Vowel	Ratio	F0 value	F1 value	F2 value	F3 value	Time
heed3	1.751592	204.1	357.5	2668.2	3429.9	542
heed2	1.858034	192.3	357.3	2719.7	3392.6	743
whod1	2.382102	140.8	335.4	856.3	2411.2	1032
whod2	2.928237	128.2	375.4	795.5	2524.7	759
whod3	2.947867	126.6	373.2	897.4	2586.4	731
heed1	3.011314	114.9	346	2818.1	3500	1170
hood2	3.382215	128.2	433.6	1018	2645.1	633
hood3	3.8088	125	476.1	1138.7	2617.4	994
heard2	3.9856	125	498.2	1317.6	1607.5	854
hid2	4.094118	119	487.2	2215	2743.9	664
hid1	4.027289	113.6	457.5	2294.6	2794.1	1291
heard3	4.234426	122	516.6	1243.7	1530.8	688
hid3	4.259786	112.4	478.8	2192.3	2929.3	605
hood1	4.290729	111.1	476.7	1089.6	2568.8	765
heard1	4.604093	112.4	517.5	1288.3	1521.2	1209
hud3	5.088	125	636	1337.3	2616.3	623
hud1	5.359415	116.3	623.3	1284.8	2670.8	923
head2	5.320432	111.1	591.1	1990	2752.9	1050
had2	5.380052	116.3	625.7	2100.4	2675.3	945
hud2	5.543422	116.3	644.7	1320.3	2589.9	602
hawed2	5.572269	119	663.1	1154.5	2709.1	916
had3	5.510351	111.1	612.2	2065.2	2599.9	806
head3	5.660019	105.3	596	1988.5	2619.2	692
head1	5.835327	108.7	634.3	1975.8	2621.6	1563
had1	5.852806	108.7	636.2	2008.5	2574.5	946
hawed3	7.112745	102	725.5	1198.5	2558.1	832

Male Talker 26

Vowel	Ratio	F0 value	F1 value	F2 value	F3 value	Time
heed2	2.098024	131.6	276.1	2121.7	2924.1	294
heed3	2.071733	140.8	291.7	2155.3	2845.3	610
heed1	2.167933	131.6	285.3	2155.7	2953.5	525
whod2	2.353285	137	322.4	960.7	2159	588
whod1	2.405101	133.3	320.6	817.8	2167.7	679
hid2	3.396524	126.6	430	1933.7	2644.9	486
heard1	3.770593	129.9	489.8	1228.8	1506.5	471
hood3	3.841185	131.6	505.5	1180.7	2403.9	673
heard3	3.865285	135.1	522.2	1308.8	1462.2	773
hood1	3.881459	131.6	510.8	1127.6	2518.7	573
hid1	3.878543	123.5	479	1842	2672.6	285
had1	3.966992	133.3	528.8	1875.8	2616.9	445
hood2	3.993522	123.5	493.2	1214.8	2403.9	560
heard2	4.016936	129.9	521.8	1152.5	1682.6	613
hud3	4.324095	129.9	561.7	1192.4	2536.9	586
hud2	4.592764	129.9	596.6	1229.9	2569.9	750
hud1	4.836626	131.6	636.5	1169.6	2604.4	599
had3	5.022672	123.5	620.3	1758	2386	667
head3	5.28278	126.6	668.8	1590	2457.9	510
head1	5.546603	126.6	702.2	1630.6	2435.8	583
hawed3	5.540249	120.5	667.6	1036.7	2512.7	708
hawed2	5.719969	128.2	733.3	1041.6	2589.4	661
head2	6.056075	117.7	712.8	1573.3	2467.5	406
hawed1	6.594118	119	784.7	1047	2545.6	346

Appendix B shows the displays of each of the 9 vowels used in the experiments produced by Talker 1. These displays are between 20 to 30 ms around the point in time that was used for the measurements. Images similar to this were used to identify vowels in perceptual experiments involving only visual inspection of the vowel (Stokes, 1996, 2001). Displays like this also led to the model of vowel perception and production introduced here.

Image 1
Talker1 Heed 1 production
570ms to 599ms

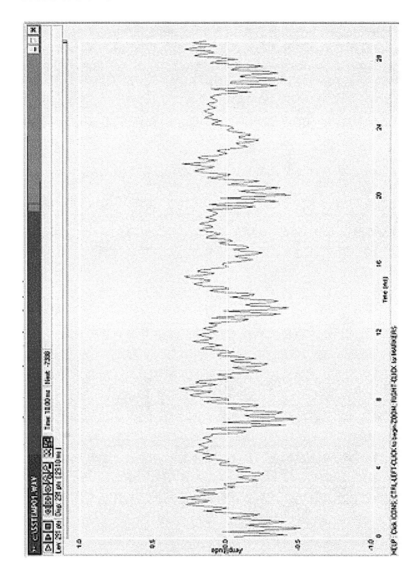

Image 2
Talker1 Whod 1 production
388ms to 411ms

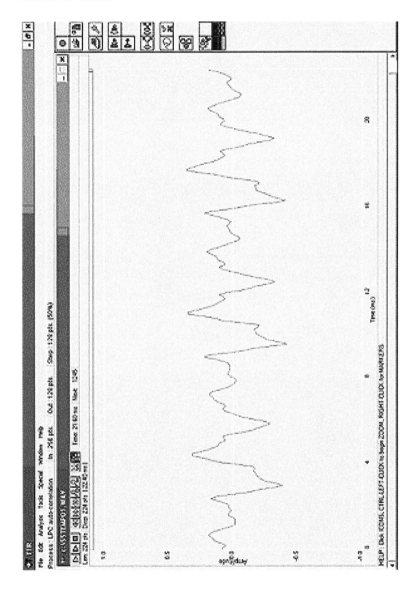

Image 3
Talker1 Hid 1 production
343ms to 365ms

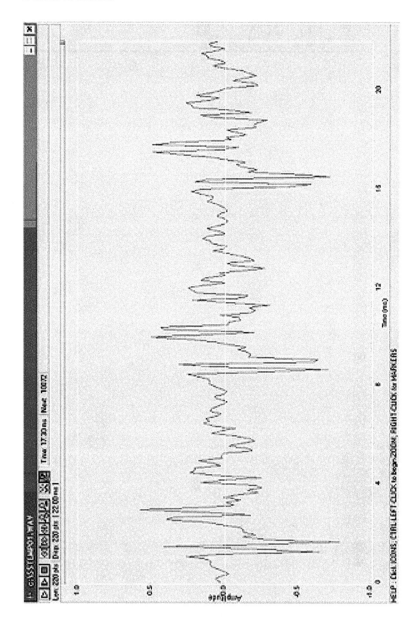

Image 4
Talker1 Hood 1 production
243ms to 265ms

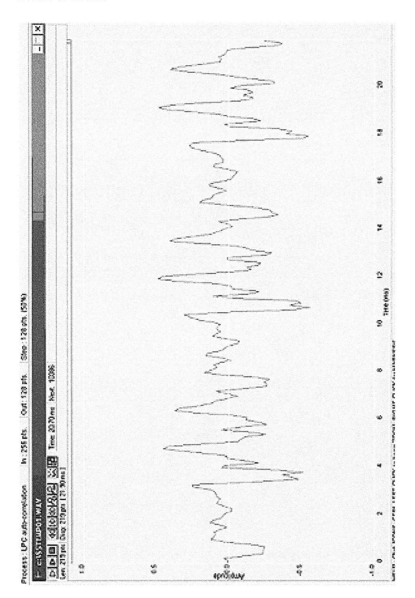

Image 5
Talker1 Had 1 production
638ms to 667ms

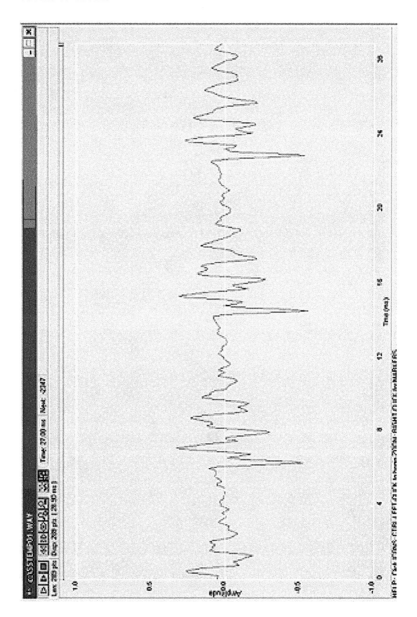

Image 6
Talker1 Head 1 production
362ms to 391ms

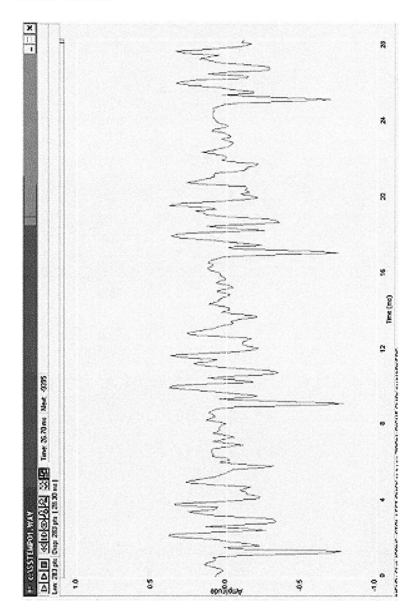

Image 7
Talker1 Hawed 1 production
441ms to 476ms

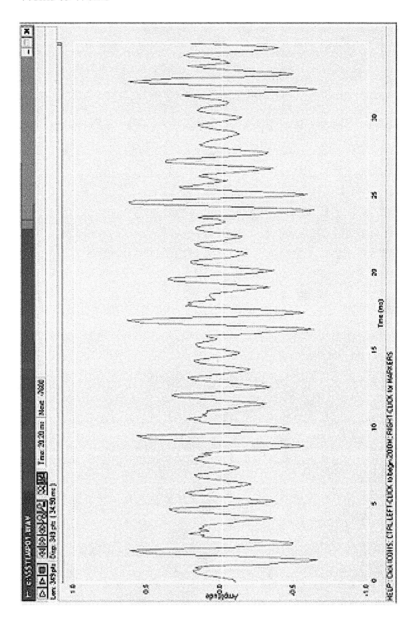

Image 8
Talker1 Hud 1 production
453ms to 482ms

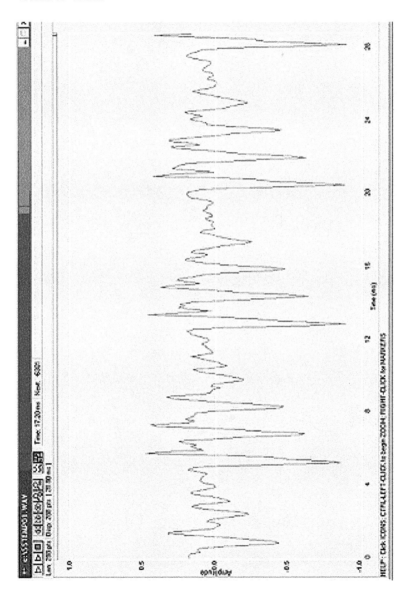

Image 9
Talker1 Heard 1 production
722ms to 748ms

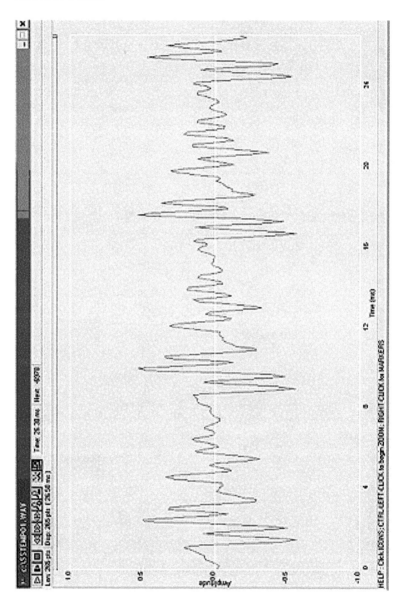

www.ingramcontent.com/pod-product-compliance
Lightning Source LLC
Chambersburg PA
CBHW070848070326
40690CB00009B/1755